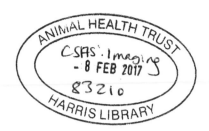

D1357192

Congenital Abnormalities of the Skull, Vertebral Column, and Central Nervous System

Editor

CURTIS W. DEWEY

VETERINARY CLINICS OF NORTH AMERICA: SMALL ANIMAL PRACTICE

www.vetsmall.theclinics.com

March 2016 • Volume 46 • Number 2

ELSEVIER

1600 John F. Kennedy Boulevard ● Suite 1800 ● Philadelphia, Pennsylvania, 19103-2899
http://www.vetsmall.theclinics.com

VETERINARY CLINICS OF NORTH AMERICA: SMALL ANIMAL PRACTICE Volume 46, Number 2
March 2016 ISSN 0195-5616, ISBN-13: 978-0-323-41671-9

Editor: Patrick Manley
Developmental Editor: Meredith Clinton

Veterinary Clinics of North America: Small Animal Practice (ISSN 0195-5616) is published bimonthly by Elsevier Inc., 360 Park Avenue South, New York, NY 10010-1710. Months of issue are January, March, May, July, September, and November. Business and Editorial Offices: 1600 John F. Kennedy Blvd., Ste. 1800, Philadelphia, PA 19103-2899. Customer Service Office: 3251 Riverport Lane, Maryland Heights, MO 63043. Periodicals postage paid at New York, NY and additional mailing offices. Subscription prices are $310.00 per year (domestic individuals), $564.00 per year (domestic institutions), $100.00 per year (domestic students/residents), $410.00 per year (Canadian individuals), $701.00 per year (Canadian institutions), $455.00 per year (international individuals), $701.00 per year (international institutions), and $220.00 per year (international and Canadian students/residents). To receive student/resident rate, orders must be accompanied by name of affiliated institution, date of term, and the *signature* of program/residency coordinator on institution letterhead. Orders will be billed at individual rate until proof of status is received. Foreign air speed delivery is included in all *Clinics* subscription prices. All prices are subject to change without notice. **POSTMASTER:** Send address changes to *Veterinary Clinics of North America: Small Animal Practice*, Elsevier Health Sciences Division, Subscription Customer Service, 3251 Riverport Lane, Maryland Heights, MO 63043. Customer Service (orders, claims, online, change of address): Elsevier Periodicals Customer Service, Elsevier Health Sciences Division Subscription **Customer Service 3251 Riverport Lane Maryland Heights, MO 63043. Tel: 1-800-654-2452 (U.S. and Canada); 314-447-8871 (outside U.S. and Canada). Fax: 314-447-8029. E-mail: journalscustomerservice-usa@elsevier.com (for print support); journalsonlinesupport-usa@elsevier.com (for online support).**

Reprints. For copies of 100 or more of articles in this publication, please contact the Commercial Reprints Department, Elsevier Inc., 360 Park Avenue South, New York, NY 10010-1710. Tel.: 212-633-3874; Fax: 212-633-3820; E-mail: reprints@elsevier.com.

Veterinary Clinics of North America: Small Animal Practice is also published in Japanese by Inter Zoo Publishing Co., Ltd., Aoyama Crystal-Bldg 5F, 3-5-12 Kitaaoyama, Minato-ku, Tokyo 107-0061, Japan.

Veterinary Clinics of North America: Small Animal Practice is covered in *Current Contents/Agriculture, Biology and Environmental Sciences, Science Citation Index, ASCA, MEDLINE/PubMed (Index Medicus), Excerpta Medica,* and *BIOSIS.*

Contributors

EDITOR

CURTIS W. DEWEY, DVM, MS
Diplomate, American College of Veterinary Internal Medicine (Neurology); Diplomate, American College of Veterinary Surgeons; Certified Veterinary Acupuncturist; Associate Professor and Section Chief, Neurology/Neurosurgery Section, Department of Clinical Sciences, Cornell University Hospital for Animals, College of Veterinary Medicine, Cornell University, Ithaca, New York

AUTHORS

JENNIFER L. BOUMA, VMD
Diplomate, American College of Veterinary Radiology; Veterinary Specialists and Emergency Services, Rochester, New York

LAURIE B. COOK, DVM
Diplomate, American College of Veterinary Internal Medicine (Neurology); Department of Veterinary Clinical Sciences, College of Veterinary Medicine, The Ohio State University, Columbus, Ohio

RONALDO C. DA COSTA, DMV, MSc, PhD
Diplomate, American College of Veterinary Internal Medicine (Neurology); Department of Veterinary Clinical Sciences, College of Veterinary Medicine, The Ohio State University, Columbus, Ohio

EMMA DAVIES, BVSc, MSc
Diplomate, European College of Veterinary Neurology; Senior Lecturer, Neurology/ Neurosurgery Section, Department of Clinical Sciences, Cornell University Hospital for Animals, College of Veterinary Medicine, Cornell University, Ithaca, New York

ALEXANDER DE LAHUNTA, DVM, PhD
Diplomate, American College of Veterinary Internal Medicine (Neurology); Diplomate, American College of Veterinary Pathology (Hon); James Law Professor of Anatomy Emeritus, College of Veterinary Medicine, Cornell University, Ithaca, New York; Rye, New Hampshire

CURTIS W. DEWEY, DVM, MS
Diplomate, American College of Veterinary Internal Medicine (Neurology); Diplomate, American College of Veterinary Surgeons; Certified Veterinary Acupuncturist; Associate Professor and Section Chief, Neurology/Neurosurgery Section, Department of Clinical Sciences, Cornell University Hospital for Animals, College of Veterinary Medicine, Cornell University, Ithaca, New York

CHELSIE M. ESTEY, MSc, DVM
Upstate Veterinary Specialties, Latham, New York

ERIC N. GLASS, DVM, MS
Diplomate, American College of Veterinary Internal Medicine (Neurology); Head of Neurology and Neurosurgery, Veterinary Specialists of North America; Section Head, Department of Neurology and Neurosurgery, Red Bank Veterinary Hospital, Tinton Falls, New Jersey

JILL HICKS, DVM
Department of Small Animal Medicine and Surgery, College of Veterinary Medicine, University of Georgia, Athens, Georgia

MARC KENT, DVM
Diplomate, American College of Veterinary Internal Medicine (Internal Medicine and Neurology); Professor, Department of Small Animal Medicine and Surgery, College of Veterinary Medicine, University of Georgia, Athens, Georgia

CATHERINE A. LOUGHIN, DVM
Diplomate, American College of Veterinary Surgeons; Diplomate, American College of Clinical Thermology; Department of Surgery, Canine Chiari Institute, Long Island Veterinary Specialists, Plainview, New York

DOMINIC J. MARINO, DVM, CCRP
Diplomate, American College of Veterinary Surgeons; Diplomate, American College of Clinical Thermology; Department of Surgery, Canine Chiari Institute, Long Island Veterinary Specialists, Plainview, New York

LARA MATIASEK, DrMedVet, MRCVS
Diplomate, European College of Veterinary Neurology; Neurology Referral Service, Tierklinik Haar, Haar, Germany

SIMON PLATT, BVM&S, MRCVS
Diplomate, American College of Veterinary Internal Medicine (Neurology); Diplomate, European College of Veterinary Neurology; Professor, Neurology and Neurosurgery Service, Department of Small Animal Medicine and Surgery, College of Veterinary Medicine, University of Georgia, Athens, Georgia

MEGHAN C. SLANINA, DVM
Neurology and Neurosurgery Resident, Department of Clinical Sciences, Cornell University Hospital for Animals, College of Veterinary Medicine, Cornell University, Ithaca, New York

RACHEL B. SONG, VMD, MS
Department of Neurology and Neurosurgery, Red Bank Veterinary Hospital, Tinton Falls, New Jersey

Contents

Ultimately, it is only with an understanding of normal embryologic development that there can be an understanding of why and how a specific malformation develops. Knowing where and when a specific part of the nervous system develops and what morphogens are at play will enable us to identify undescribed malformation, as well as better define causality. The following article reviews the normal embryologic development of the mammalian nervous system and is intended to serve as a foundation for understanding the various malformations presented in this issue.

There are several types of hydrocephalus, which are characterized based on the location of the cerebrospinal fluid (CSF) accumulation. Physical features of animals with congenital hydrocephalus may include a dome-shaped skull, persistent fontanelle, and bilateral ventrolateral strabismus. Medical therapy involves decreasing the production of CSF. The most common surgical treatment is placement of a ventriculoperitoneal shunt. Postoperative complications may include infection, blockage, drainage abnormalities, and mechanical failure.

Chiari-like malformation is a condition of the craniocervical junction in which there is a mismatch of the structures of the caudal cranial fossa causing the cerebellum to herniate into the foramen magnum. This herniation can lead to fluid buildup in the spinal cord, also known as syringomyelia. Pain is the most common clinical sign followed by scratching. Other neurologic signs noted are facial nerve deficits, seizures, vestibular syndrome, ataxia, menace deficit, proprioceptive deficits, head tremor, temporal muscle atrophy, and multifocal central nervous system signs. MRI is the diagnostic of choice, but computed tomography can also be used.

The term craniocervical junction abnormality (CJA) is an umbrella term for a variety of malformations that occur in the craniocervical region. These abnormalities include Chiari-like malformation, atlantooccipital overlapping,

juvenile and adult small breed dogs. These anomalous vertebrae typically result in various degrees of kyphosis and scoliosis in the region of the abnormality. They are thought to occur following developmental errors during embryonic or fetal vertebral segmentation and ossification; most are incidental. This article focuses on those anomalies of the thoracic vertebral bodies that lead to clinical signs of neurologic dysfunction. Based on a limited number of reported cases, the prognosis for surgically managed dogs with thoracic vertebral body abnormalities is favorable.

Jennifer L. Bouma

Articular process anomalies are considered congenital. Their occurrence in specific breeds may be indicative of undetermined genetics. Clinical significance varies and is interdependent upon location, function and anatomy. Etiology, uniform nomenclature and classification of vertebral articular process anomalies in the dog are lacking; however, recent efforts are beginning to address this deficit. This author proposes that the term *articular process dysplasia* appropriately encompasses the spectrum of anomalies in severity as well as including those affecting both the cranial and caudal articular processes. The general category description of *articular process dypslasia* doesn't preclude, but rather allows for more specific designations.

Rachel B. Song, Eric N. Glass, and Marc Kent

Spina bifida, with or without meningocele, or meningomyelocele, is encountered infrequently in small animal practice. The English bulldog and Manx cat are breeds that are predisposed. Although often silent, in those animals with clinical signs it is important to recognize the signs early and to understand the appropriate imaging modalities employed in establishing a diagnosis. In a select population of affected animals, proposed surgical intervention may be considered to prevent neurologic decline, prevent secondary complications, and potentially improve outcomes.

VETERINARY CLINICS OF NORTH AMERICA: SMALL ANIMAL PRACTICE

RELATED INTEREST

Veterinary Clinics of North America: Exotic Animal Practice
January 2016, Volume 19, Issue 1
Soft Tissue Surgery
Kurt K. Sladky and Christoph Mans, *Editors*

THE CLINICS ARE NOW AVAILABLE ONLINE!
Access your subscription at:
www.theclinics.com

Preface

Congenital Malformations of the Skull, Vertebral Column, and Central Nervous System

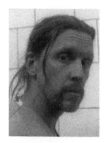

Curtis W. Dewey, DVM, MS
Editor

This issue of the *Veterinary Clinics of North America: Small Animal Practice* is meant to provide the practicing clinician with an overview of the more commonly encountered congenital abnormalities affecting the central nervous system, as well as various diagnostic and therapeutic options available for these disorders. As is often the case with this sort of amalgamation of topics, there exists some degree of controversy regarding these disorders, especially surrounding what constitutes appropriate treatment. Controversy is not necessarily a negative thing, though. Tupac Shakur once stated, "out of controversy comes conversation, out of conversation comes action." This is actually a partial quotation. The first part of this quotation described controversy as being a product of anger. Although I doubt many veterinarians become angry over the diseases described in the following pages, I feel that the complexity and severity of many of the disorders covered in this issue can lead to frustration for both the clinician and the pet owner. As you will learn (if you don't know this already) by reading through these articles, many of these disorders are still a source of frustration, even though progress has been made in their diagnosis and treatment over the years. Fortunately, we have made tremendous progress in our understanding of these congenital problems, as reflected in the voluminous original research publications over the last decade. We still have a lot of work to accomplish, but things have come a long way in a very short period of time. My hope is that this issue will—in addition to serving as a general information source—be useful as a springboard for further conversation among clinicians, conversation that will lead to action for the benefit of our patients.

I would like to thank all of the contributing authors of this issue for putting in so much hard work. I also would like to thank everyone involved at Elsevier for their attention to detail and their patience with me, especially Patrick Manley and Meredith Clinton. Finally, I want to thank my awesome wife, Janette, and our six fantastic children

http://dx.doi.org/10.1016/j.cvsm.2015.12.002
0195-5616/16/$ – see front matter © 2016 Published by Elsevier Inc.
vetsmall.theclinics.com

(Jordan, Isaiah, Ethan, Carver, Solé, and Jolie) for putting up with my complaints (more than the average level) of having way too much to do while this compilation was being created.

Curtis W. Dewey, DVM, MS
Department of Clinical Sciences
College of Veterinary Medicine
Cornell University
T6 002C Vet Research Tower
Ithaca, NY 14853, USA

E-mail address:
cwd27@cornell.edu

Embryonic Development of the Central Nervous System

Alexander de Lahunta, DVM, PhD[a],*, Eric N. Glass, DVM, MS[b], Marc Kent, DVM[c]

KEYWORDS

- Embryonic development • Central nervous system • Mammalian nervous system

KEY POINTS

- Clinical neurology is founded on the understanding of the interplay between the anatomic structure of the nervous system and its function.
- MRI provides the modern veterinary neurologist with an unparalleled tool in which the structure of the nervous system can be investigated.
- For congenital malformations of the nervous system, vertebrae, and cranium, the diagnosis has been based on pattern recognition.
- The complex orchestration of the normal development of the nervous system requires that these tissues be present at specific times and in a specific differentiated state.
- This delicately timed process involves a plethora of morphogens that also need be present at specific sites and times.

INTRODUCTION

Unquestionably, clinical neurology is founded on the understanding of the interplay between the anatomic structure of the nervous system and its function. MRI provides the modern veterinary neurologist with an unparalleled tool in which the structure of the nervous system can be investigated. In the past, congenital malformations of the nervous system, vertebrae, and cranium were relegated, for the most part, to postmortem examinations. Today, MRI allows for such malformations to be identified and

The author has nothing to disclose.

This article and its figures have been adapted with permission from de Lahunta A, Glass E, Kent M. Development of the nervous system: malformation. In: de Lahunta A, Glass E, Kent M, editors. Veterinary neuroanatomy and clinical neurology. 4th edition. Philadelphia: Saunders; 2015. p. 45–66.

[a] College of Veterinary Medicine, Cornell University, PO Box 907, Rye, NH 03870, USA; [b] Department of Neurology and Neurosurgery, Red Bank Veterinary Hospital, 197 Hance Avenue, Tinton Falls, NJ 07724, USA; [c] Department of Small Animal Medicine and Surgery, College of Veterinary Medicine, University of Georgia, 2200 College Station Road, Athens, GA 30602, USA
* Corresponding author.
E-mail address: ad43@cornell.edu

Vet Clin Small Anim 46 (2016) 193–216
http://dx.doi.org/10.1016/j.cvsm.2015.10.011
0195-5616/16/$ – see front matter

explored antemortem. For many of these malformations, the diagnosis has been based on pattern recognition; to see an abnormal structure in one animal and be told what it represents allows one to make the same diagnosis the next time that same abnormality is seen in another animal. However, gaining a greater understanding of congenital malformations necessitates an in-depth knowledge of embryology. The complex orchestration of the normal development of the nervous system requires not only the presence of normal pluripotent tissues but that these tissues be present at specific times and in a specific differentiated state. Moreover, this delicately timed process involves a plethora of morphogens that also need to be present at specific sites and times. Ultimately, it is only with an understanding of normal embryologic development that there can be an understanding of why and how a specific malformation develops. Knowing from where and when a specific part of the nervous system develops and what morphogens are at play will enable us to identify undescribed malformation as well as better define causality. The following article reviews the normal embryologic development of the mammalian nervous system and is intended to serve as a foundation for the understanding of the various malformations presented in this issue.

NEURAL TUBE

Early in development, all vertebrate embryos form 3 layers or sheets of cells from which all tissues and organs in the emerging fetus will be formed. The outer or dorsal most layer is the *ectoderm*, which will form the epidermis, neural tissues, and some of the skeletal and connective tissues of the head. The deepest, innermost layer is the *endoderm*, which will form the lining of the digestive tract, the respiratory system, and organs associated with digestion. Between these two layers is a more loosely arrayed population of cells called *mesoderm*, which will form most of the muscles, skeletal tissues, the urogenital system, and the heart and blood vessels.

The central nervous system (CNS) is a tubular structure that first develops as a thickening of the ectoderm, *the neural plate*, which develops dorsal to a column of mesodermal cells called the notochord. The notochord is a longitudinal column of mesodermal cells that originates from the embryonic primitive streak and establishes the long axis of the embryo. This neural plate invaginates along its long axis, initially forming a neural groove, followed by an elevation of the lateral extremities of the original plate called *neural folds*. These folds meet centrally and fuse over the neural groove to form a *neural tube* and *neural canal*. As the neural tube forms, it separates from the non-neural ectoderm, which grows over the dorsum of the tube to fuse along the midline. As this fusion and separation of ectodermal layers occurs, a longitudinal column of ectodermal epithelial cells arises from the junction of non-neural and neural ectoderm and separates from these two structures when the neural tube is formed. These bilateral columns, situated dorsolateral to the neural tube throughout its length, are the columns of *neural crest* cells (**Fig. 1**).

Closure of the neural tube progresses rostrally and caudally from the level of the site of development of the rhombencephalon, the most caudal division of the brain. The caudal closure forms most of the spinal cord. Closure of the brain portion of the neural tube may initially occur at multiple sites and progress rostrally and caudally. The locations of these sites vary among species. Before complete closure, the most rostral opening is the *rostral neuropore* (**Fig. 2**). Similarly, the caudal opening of the neural tube is called the *caudal neuropore*. The caudal portion of the spinal cord develops from the caudal end of the closed neural tube as an extension of a column of neuroepithelial cells that grows caudally on the midline between the notochord and skin ectoderm. A cavitation within this column of cells produces an extension of the neural canal. This portion of the neural tube will

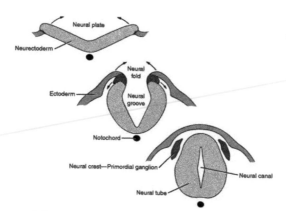

Fig. 1. Development of the neural tube, transverse sections.

ultimately form the caudal, the sacral, and a variable number of lumbar spinal cord segments. An opening may persist at the caudal end of the neural tube, allowing communication with the subarachnoid space of the leptomeninges at the conus medullaris.

The rostral end of the neural tube develops rapidly and produces 3 vesicles, from rostral to caudal: the *prosencephalon, mesencephalon,* and *rhombencephalon* (**Fig. 3**). Early in its development, the prosencephalon has lateral enlargements, the *optic vesicles,* which grow laterally to contact the overlying skin ectoderm. The neuroectoderm of these

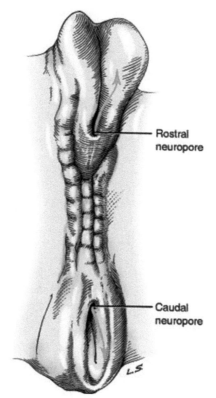

Fig. 2. Dorsal view of neural tube closure.

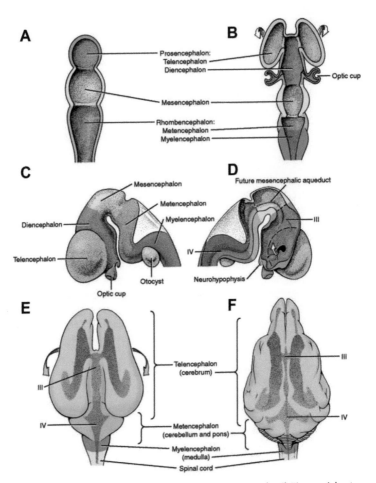

Fig. 3. Development of brain vesicles. (*A*) Three vesicle stages. (*B–F*) Five vesicle stages; III, IV: ventricles.

vesicles will form the nervous and the non-nervous layers of the retina in the eye. Two additional swellings emerge from the rostral prosencephalon and grow out of the neural tube on each side laterally and dorsally. These *telencephalic vesicles* completely overgrow the original vesicular system and form the *cerebral hemispheres*. The portion of the prosencephalon that remains at the rostral end of the neural tube is the *diencephalon*. The optic vesicles remain associated with the diencephalon. The neural canal within the diencephalon is the *third ventricle*. It communicates rostrolaterally with the neural canal of each telencephalon (cerebral hemisphere), which is the *lateral ventricle* (first and second ventricles). This small communication on each side is the *interventricular foramen*. The nuclei of the thalamus and hypothalamus develop in the diencephalon. The neurohypophysis is a ventral outgrowth of the diencephalon. The cerebral cortex and most of the basal nuclei develop in the telencephalon.

The neural canal of the *mesencephalon* is reduced to a narrow tubular space called the *mesencephalic aqueduct*.

The *rhombencephalon* gives rise to the metencephalon and myelencephalon.

From the rostral *rhombencephalon*, the *cerebellum* or dorsal metencephalon develops dorsally. The remaining ventral metencephalon becomes the *pons*. The caudal rhombencephalon forms the myelencephalon or *medulla oblongata*. The *fourth ventricle* is the lumen of the neural canal in the rhombencephalon. It communicates with the subarachnoid space that develops around the neural tube by way of openings that arise in the wall of the neural tube caudal to the developing cerebellum. These openings are called the *lateral apertures*. The neural canal continues caudally as the *central canal* of the spinal cord.

Cell Differentiation

In the first stage of development within the wall of the neural tube, the cells, which are commonly referred to as *neuroepithelial* or *neuroectodermal cells*, are organized in a pseudostratified arrangement; thus, the initial neural tube is 1 cell in thickness. The cell membrane of each cell spans the full width of the neural tube (from the external surface of neural tube to the luminal surface of the neural canal), yet the nucleus of each cell is located at various levels within each cell. These cells are all mitotically active; therefore, as the cells divide and proliferate, the thickness of the wall of the tube increases. As this occurs, the nucleus migrates within the cytoplasm of each cell; their position depends on the cell's stage of mitosis.

During interphase, the nuclei are located on the external surface of the neural tube. Chromosomal DNA duplication occurs with the nucleus in that position. As the nucleus enters mitosis, it migrates through the cytoplasm to the neural canal. The peripheral portion of the cytoplasm and the cell membrane also retract to the luminal position where cell division is completed. The two new daughter cells extend their cytoplasm and cell membranes back to the external surface of the neural tube. The nucleus migrates back to the periphery again. In this position, this cell can undergo another mitosis or it can differentiate. Because the nucleus is at the external surface during interphase, differentiation occurs at the external surface of the neural tube. Thus, in a short time a new layer of differentiating cells appears on the external surface of the actively dividing layer. The mitotic layer of cells is the *germinal layer* (also called the *ventricular zone*). The cells undergoing differentiation form the *mantle layer* (**Fig. 4**). Those located at the external surface of the neural tube are called the *marginal layer*.

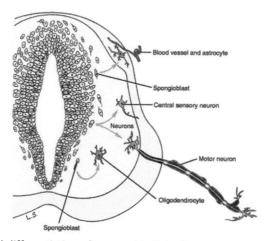

Fig. 4. Mitosis and differentiation of neuroepithelial cells.

The cells that are differentiated are of 2 types: immature neurons and spongioblasts. *Immature neurons* are the primary parenchymal cells of the nervous system. They are often referred to as neuroblasts; but this is a misnomer because once the cell differentiates into a neuron, it will not divide again as the term *neuroblast* implies. The differentiated immature neuron develops extensively, forming long processes in becoming a mature functioning cell, but it does not divide again. *Spongioblasts* are the progenitors of the neuroectodermal supporting cells of the nervous system, the *neuroglia* (glue). Two of the 3 forms of glial cells are derived from these spongioblasts: *astrocytes* and *oligodendrocytes* (see **Fig. 4**). The third glial cell is the *microglial cell*, which is mesodermal in origin. It is a monocyte that enters the nervous system from the blood supply.

As the primitive neurons and spongioblasts differentiate and grow and the neurons produce processes, the neural tube becomes arranged in 3 concentric layers (**Fig. 5**). Adjacent to the lumen of the neural tube is the *germinal layer* of proliferating neuroepithelial cells. This proliferative mitotic activity will ultimately be exhausted, reducing the germinal layer to a single layer of cells ranging from squamous to columnar and without processes. These cells are the *ependymal cells*. These ependymal cells line the entire lumen of the neural tube, which includes the ventricular system in the brain and the central canal of the spinal cord. Peripheral to this germinal layer in the embryonic neural tube is the thick layer of differentiated cells, the immature neurons, and spongioblasts. They form the *mantle layer*, which will ultimately become the gray matter of the definitive spinal cord, the nuclei of the brainstem, the nuclei and cortex of the cerebellum, and the basal nuclei and cerebral cortex of the telencephalon. This 3-layered relationship persists in the developing spinal cord. The initial external layer of the neural tube is the *marginal layer*; it is initially composed primarily of the growing axonal processes of the neuronal cell bodies in the mantle layer. These axons will be myelinated by the oligodendroglial cells forming tracts in the white matter. In contrast, in the telencephalon, there is a migration of neurons from the mantle layer to the external surface of the marginal layer of the neural tube. This migration gives rise to the overlying gray matter of the cerebral cortex in the telencephalon as this structure develops.

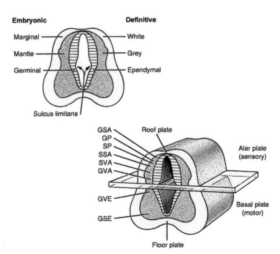

Fig. 5. Functional organization of the neural tube. GP, general proprioception; GSA, general somatic afferent; GSE, general somatic efferent; GVA, general visceral afferent; GVE, general visceral efferent; SP, special proprioception; SSA, special somatic afferent; SVA, special visceral afferent.

From the mesencephalon caudally, a longitudinal groove, the *sulcus limitans*, appears in the lateral wall of the neural canal. Thus, the neural canal can be artificially divided into dorsal and ventral portions by an imaginary dorsal plane at the level of this sulcus. The dorsal portion is called the *alar plate* and the ventral portion the *basal plate*. Functionally, the alar plate mantle layer is concerned predominantly with sensory systems and the basal plate mantle layer with motor systems (see **Fig. 5**).

NEUROGENESIS

Having established the role of the neural tube in the initial development of the CNS, it is appropriate to consider neurogenesis in the adult animal. It is recognized that once a primitive neuron is differentiated in the neural tube mantle layer, that cell will not undergo mitosis again and the mature neuron will persist for the life of the animal. The premise is that once the CNS is formed, neurogenesis ceases to occur. If a population of neurons is lost because of disease or injury, those neurons are not replaced.

Although a finite time in development exists for most neurogenesis, substantial research supports *selective postnatal neurogenesis* throughout the life of the animal. In the embryonic neural tube, the embryonic neuroepithelial cells give rise to a cell line referred to as *radial glia*. During development, these radial glia function to guide the developing primitive neurons to their sites of destination in the neural tube, such as the cerebral cortex. However, in addition, it is now recognized that these radial glia may also differentiate into primitive neurons, astrocytes, oligodendrocytes, and ependymal cells. After development is completed, the undifferentiated radial glial cells populate the subventricular zone, which is most evident rostrally in association with the lateral ventricle of the frontal lobe. Here, these radial astrocytes function as neuronal stem cells as well as a source of astrocytes and oligodendrocytes. This adult neurogenesis occurs primarily in the rostral cerebral subventricular zone, where the newly formed neurons populate the olfactory bulb. The other site is the subgranular zone of the hippocampal dentate gyrus, where they serve to replace dentate gyrus granule neurons. The activated neuronal stem cells at these sites are derived from a unique population of radial glia that is adjacent to the ependymal cells at these sites. The function of these cells formed in adult neurogenesis both in the subventricular and subgranular zones needs further study with regard to their purpose in mammals. These subventricular zone adult neuronal stem cells are thought to be the source of some of the gliomas that occur in the brains of humans and domestic animals. It is also thought that these cells may play some role in plasticity after injury. Additionally, it is hoped that these cells may be harvested for cell replacement after devastating injury to the CNS or neurodegenerative processes.

MEDULLA SPINALIS: SPINAL CORD

In this article, the term *spinal cord* is used rather than medulla spinalis, the nomenclature preferred by the *Nomina Anatomica Veterinaria*. The spinal cord is contained within the vertebral column. A common error in nomenclature is to refer to the vertebral column as the spine. This reference is inappropriate as the spine is a process of the vertebral arch. The development of the nervous system depends on complex genetic factors. Two signaling centers have been recognized as being responsible for the development of the spinal cord portion of the neural tube. One is the surface ectoderm adjacent to the neuroectoderm that formed the neural plate. These surface ectodermal cells secrete *bone morphogenetic protein 4* (BMP-4), a cytokine that enters the neural tube and directs the development of the dorsal portion of the neural tube. BMP-4 is responsible for triggering the secretion of *transforming growth factor beta*, which diffuses ventrally in the neural tube where it is responsible for the formation of dorsal horn neurons. The second signaling center is the notochord and cells within the basal plate and their secretory signaling molecule, *Sonic hedgehog* (SHH). SHH diffuses dorsally into the neural tube and is responsible for directing the development of the ventral portion of the neural tube with its ventral horn neurons.

The spinal cord provides the least complicated example of the symmetric development of the neural tube by layers. Ventral growth of the two mantle layer basal plates and associated marginal layers beyond the level of the floor plate (see **Figs. 3–5; Fig. 6**) leaves a separation between the two sides, which is the *ventral median fissure*. The mantle and marginal layers of the alar plates grow dorsally. The dorsal marginal layers fuse on the median plane to form a *dorsal median septum* that may be poorly defined. The external margin of this septum forms the *dorsal median sulcus*. This midline growth displaces the roof plate region ventrally, resulting in a reduction of the neural canal to form the small *central canal* of the spinal cord lined by ependymal cells. The mantle layer of the alar plate becomes the *dorsal gray column* (also referred to as *horn*), and that of the basal plate becomes the *ventral gray column*. The mantle zone at the plane of the sulcus limitans becomes the *intermediate gray column* (see **Fig. 6**).

Not only is there a gross topographic differentiation of function of primitive neurons between the alar and basal plates but within the mantle layer of each plate, neurons are further arranged in functional columns. The *general visceral afferent* and *general visceral efferent* (GVE) neurons are located adjacent to each other in their respective gray columns on either side of the dorsal plane through the sulcus limitans. The *general somatic afferent* (GSA) and *general proprioceptive* neuronal columns are located dorsally in the alar plate of the mantle layer, and the *general somatic efferent* (GSE) column is located ventrally in the basal plate of the mantle layer. Because the relative size of the components of each spinal cord segment depends on the volume of tissue being innervated, at the levels of the limbs the spinal cord segments

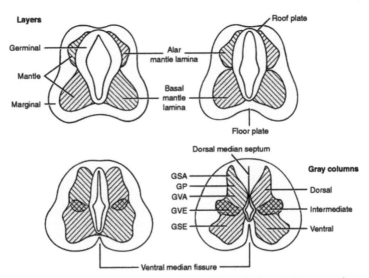

Fig. 6. Development and functional organization of the spinal cord. GP, general proprioception; GSA, general somatic afferent; GSE, general somatic efferent; GVA, general visceral afferent; GVE, general visceral efferent.

responsible for their innervation are enlarged forming the cervical and lumbosacral *intumescences*. The ultimate growth to maturity of a neuron in the peripheral nervous system depends on its appropriate innervation of a muscle cell (GSE) or formation of a peripheral receptor (GSA, general proprioception [GP]). The lack of such innervation results in the degeneration of that neuron. In the cervical and thoracolumbar regions where appendages are not innervated, the immature primitive neurons in the basal plate mantle layer and the adjacent spinal ganglion that fail to innervate structures will degenerate by a process of cell death referred to as *apoptosis*. The shape of the ventral gray column depicts the results of this process.

In the spinal cord basal plate mantle layer, the GSE neurons located medially innervate the axial skeletal muscles. Those located laterally innervate the appendicular skeletal muscles. Within these areas of the ventral gray column, the GSE neuronal cell bodies can be further grouped according to the specific nerve that contains their axon and by the specific muscles innervated.

The growth of axons of the basal plate neurons through the marginal layer and outside the neural tube forms the *ventral root* and part of the spinal nerve and further branching of the nerves as they extend to the muscles that they innervate. This branching includes the GSE neurons located in the ventral gray column and the GVE neurons located in the intermediate gray column adjacent to the sulcus limitans. These latter GVE neurons are the preganglionic lower motor neurons of the autonomic nervous system. This intermediate gray column is only present in the thoracic, cranial lumbar, and sacral spinal cord segments. In the other segments, it was present in the embryo but subsequently degenerated because of the absence of a target organ or biochemical attractant. These GVE neurons terminate in ganglia in the peripheral nervous system that contain cell bodies of the postganglionic axons in this 2-neuron lower motor neuron system (see also **Fig. 6**; **Figs. 7** and **8**).

Neural Crest

At the junction of neural plate and surface ectoderm, BMP and WNT protein induce the ectodermal cells to develop mesenchymal features, penetrate the ectodermal basal lamina, and form a column of cells dorsolateral to the neural tube. This bilateral column extends the full length of the neural tube and is referred to as the *neural crest*. These two columns of neural crest cells become segmented adjacent to each somite and developing spinal cord segment to provide the neurons that form the *spinal ganglia* at each segment (see **Figs. 1** and **7**). One portion of the axon that emerges from each of these cell bodies grows centrally into the spinal cord segment to enter the alar plate dorsal gray column forming the *dorsal root*. The other portion of the axon grows distally to form a sensory component of the spinal nerve and its further branches. The point of penetration of the marginal white matter layer of the spinal cord segment by the axons in the dorsal and ventral roots divides the spinal cord white matter processes into 3 regions called *funiculi*. These funiculi are the dorsal, lateral, and ventral funiculi on each side of the spinal cord.

The formation of spinal ganglia is only one of many outcomes of neural crest differentiation. Before its segregation into spinal ganglia, an early migration of cells from this neural crest column provides melanoblasts to the somitic dermatome and adjacent epidermis as well as the ganglionic neurons in the 2-neuron GVE system of the autonomic nervous system.

These latter cell bodies form the ganglia of the sympathetic trunk and the abdominal plexus sympathetic ganglia as well as the medullary cells in the adrenal gland (see **Fig. 8**). These adrenal medullary cells do not grow any processes but synthesize and elaborate into the blood stream the same endocrine substance, norepinephrine, that

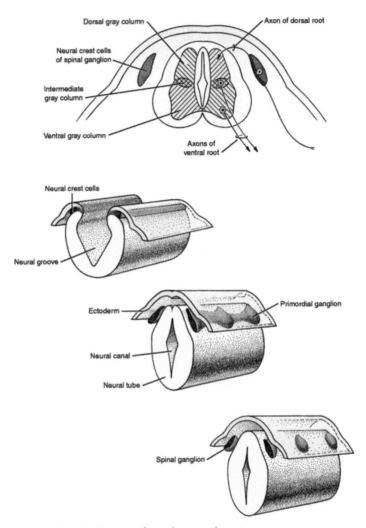

Fig. 7. Spinal ganglia development from the neural crest.

is the neurotransmitter released at the telodendron of the sympathetic postganglionic axon derived from the neural crest cells. Although the melanoblasts and GVE neurons seem unrelated, their common denominator is the unique metabolism of tyrosine, which provides melanin for the melanocytes and norepinephrine for the neuron. In addition, there is extensive migration of the neural crest cells into the wall of the developing gastrointestinal tract. These cells will form the ganglionic neurons of the parasympathetic portion of the GVE lower motor neuron as well as interneurons; they form the glial cells that develop in the wall of the bowel, creating what is referred to as the *enteric nervous system*. The latter is extremely extensive, complex, and presumably is entirely derived from the neural crest cells. A similar migration forms the ganglionic parasympathetic neurons for the urogenital system. In addition to these nervous system structures, the neural crest contributes to the formation of bone and cartilage in the skull and derivatives of the branchial arches; to the wall of the great vessels at the base of

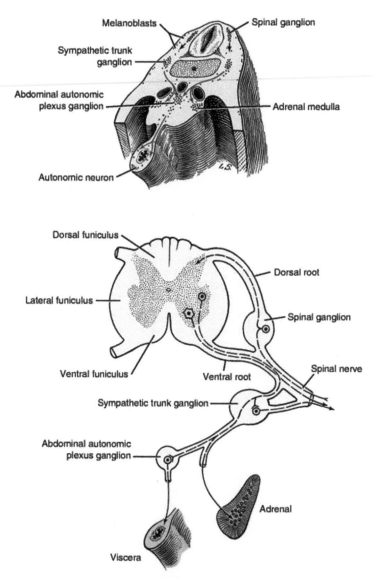

Fig. 8. Neural crest contribution to the development of GVE neurons.

the heart; and to thyroid parafollicular (C) cells, odontoblasts, a portion of the leptomeninges and the lemmocytes, Schwann cells, that form the myelin of the peripheral nervous system. This diversity is an amazing display of developmental capabilities in an initial column of cells.

Many studies have and are continuing to contribute to our understanding of the molecular basis for brain development. Signals derived from homeobox genes are expressed in the notochord, prechordal plate, and the rostral neural plate, which influence the regional specialization of the brain into its prosencephalic, mesencephalic, and rhombencephalic divisions. As in the development of the spinal cord, the signaling protein SHH, secreted by the prechordal plate and the rostral notochord, influences the ventral patterning of the brain, and BMP-4 and BMP-7, secreted by the adjacent surface ectoderm, control the dorsal patterning of the brain.

MYELENCEPHALON: MEDULLA OBLONGATA

In this article, the term *medulla oblongata* is shortened to *medulla*. The medulla is the most caudal portion of the brainstem and is continuous caudally with the spinal cord. The *brainstem* includes the diencephalon, mesencephalon, ventral metencephalon, and myelencephalon. It is the stem on which are located the cerebellum and cerebrum.

The basic formation of the medulla involves only a slight modification of the development described for the spinal cord. The narrow mid-dorsal roof plate of the initial neural tube (see **Figs. 5** and **6**) is stretched extensively instead of being obliterated by the proliferating alar plate and marginal tissue as it is in the spinal cord. Imagine grasping the midline roof plate of the neural tube with both hands and then pulling your hands apart, sideways. This pulling would stretch out a thin layer of neural tube (roof plate) and displace the entire alar and basal plates to a lateral and ventral position (**Fig. 9**). This displacement would enlarge the neural canal to form the *fourth ventricle* of the medulla, which is covered dorsally by only a single cell layer of neuroepithelial cells. At this site, these cells will not enter mitosis but will remain as a single layer of ependymal cells. The sulcus limitans that is present on the ventrolateral wall of the fourth ventricle provides the plane of division of the medulla into a ventromedial basal plate and a dorsolateral alar plate, which have the same functional significance as in the spinal cord development (see **Fig. 9**).

Throughout the brainstem, the mantle layer of the neural tube is broken up into *nuclei* that are collections of neuronal cell bodies with a common purpose, and they are interspersed with neuronal processes. Some nuclei are more distinct than others. The functional columns described in the spinal cord have a similar location in the brainstem. In addition, there are neurons in the medulla that are organized into functional groups that are present in cranial nerves VI through XII (see **Fig. 9**).

In domestic animals, cranial nerves VI through XII and the trapezoid body are part of the medulla. The rostral border of the medulla is the caudal border of the pontine transverse fibers. In primates and some nondomesticated species, the transverse fibers of the pons expand caudally to cover the trapezoid body, so cranial nerves VI through VIII are included with V in the pons. Cranial nerves VI, VII, IX, X, XI, and XII contain general somatic efferent neurons. The medullary nuclei of cranial nerves VI and XII are located in an interrupted column along the median plane adjacent to the fourth ventricle. The *hypoglossal nucleus* is very long. The GSE neuronal cell bodies of the facial nerve have migrated from their initial formation in the mantle layer to form the *facial nucleus* in a ventrolateral position, which is closer to their common source of sensory stimuli coursing into the medulla in the spinal tract of the trigeminal nerve and the adjacent nucleus of the spinal tract of the trigeminal nerve. This phenomenon of migration is referred to as *neurobiotaxis*. As a result of this migration, the axons leaving this facial nucleus initially course dorsomedially to the floor of the fourth ventricle before turning to course ventrolaterally to leave the medulla and form the facial nerve. This migration is in part regulated by T-box transcription factor, Tbx20; the final migration of the neurons is under control of oligo2 function. The GSE cell bodies of cranial nerves IX, X, and XI undergo a similar migration ventrolaterally and accumulate in the *nucleus ambiguus*, which is well named because it is a poorly defined nucleus. The preganglionic neurons of the parasympathetic portion of the GVE system are located in an interrupted column

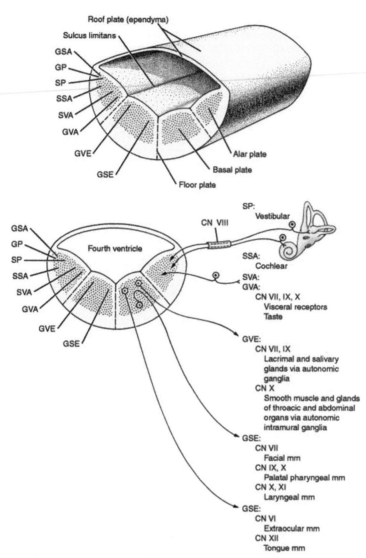

Fig. 9. Functional organization of cranial nerves (CNs) VI to XII in the myelencephalon. CN VI, abducent; CN VII, facial; CN VIII, vestibulocochlear; CN IX, glossopharyngeal; CN X, vagus; CN XI, accessory; CN XII, hypoglossal; GVA, general visceral afferent; SP, special proprioception; SSA, special somatic afferent; SVA, special visceral afferent.

just ventromedial to the sulcus limitans, which is comparable with the intermediate gray column cell bodies in the spinal cord. Their axons leave the medulla in cranial nerves VII, IX, X, and XI.

The sensory components of cranial nerves associated with the medulla arise primarily from primitive neurons that develop from the column of neural crest cells, with a few arising from ectodermal cells that proliferate from branchial arch ectoderm. The latter areas are referred to as cranial *placodes*. These two sources form the sensory ganglia of cranial nerves VII, IX, and X, which are concerned with general visceral afferent and special visceral afferent (taste) function. Ectodermal cells derived from the *otic placode* form the sensory ganglia of cranial nerve VIII, which is concerned with special proprioception for vestibular system function and with the special somatic afferent system for auditory function. These cranial nerve VIII ganglia are located in the inner ear within the petrosal portion of the temporal bone. Their axons course into the alar plate region of the medulla to synapse on cell bodies comparable with the dorsal gray column cell bodies in the spinal cord (see **Fig. 9**).

The leptomeninges that surround the entire developing CNS (neural tube) arise from neural crest cells and adjacent mesodermal cells. These meninges contain the bulk of the blood vessels that supply the CNS and the roots of cranial and spinal nerves. The roof plate of ependymal cells that covers the fourth ventricle and the thin layer of vascularized pia associated with it is called the *tela choroidea* of the fourth ventricle. The capillary blood vessels in this tela choroidea proliferate to form the 2 longitudinal rows of a dense capillary bed. The adjacent ependymal cells enlarge into cuboidal cells, and the entire structure (cuboidal ependymal cells, pia mater, and capillary bed) protrudes into the lumen of the fourth ventricle (**Fig. 10**). This structure is called

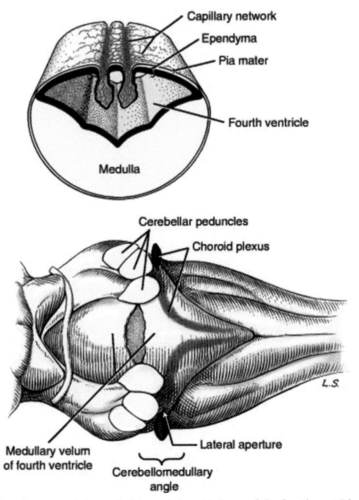

Fig. 10. Development of the roof plate and choroid plexus of the fourth ventricle.

the *choroid plexus* of the fourth ventricle. By strict definition, only the proliferated capillary bed is the plexus. Thus, the choroid plexus of the fourth ventricle comprises 2 sagittal lines parallel to and on either side of the median plane. These lines extend rostrally from the caudal part of the fourth ventricle to the level of the cerebellar peduncles where each plexus turns laterally. At this point there is an opening that develops in the medullary roof plate, called the *lateral aperture*. This aperture allows communication between the lumen of the fourth ventricle and the subarachnoid space that develops in the leptomeninges. At the level of this lateral aperture, the choroid plexus protrudes from the lumen of the fourth ventricle out through the aperture, where it is visible on each side at the cerebellomedullary angle (see **Fig. 10**). The aperture itself is invisible grossly because it is filled with this choroid plexus. The choroid plexus is visible here during intracranial surgery as well as on T1-weighted postcontrast MR images. The choroid plexus is a major site of formation of cerebrospinal fluid. In domestic animals, the lateral aperture is the only communication between the ventricular system of the brain and the subarachnoid space, which makes it critical for the maintenance of normal intracranial pressure. Primates have an additional aperture, the median aperture, located caudally on the median plane in the caudal medullary velum of the fourth ventricle, which is termed the *foramen of Magendie*, an eponym that is unnecessary to learn for our veterinary patients.

METENCEPHALON: CEREBELLUM AND PONS

The initial development of the metencephalon is comparable with that of the myelencephalon. *Cranial nerve V, the trigeminal nerve*, is associated with this segment of the brainstem (**Fig. 11**). Its motor neurons arise in the basal plate mantle layer, migrate a short way ventrolaterally into the parenchyma of the pons, and form a small, well-defined motor nucleus. These neurons function in the GSE system and innervate the muscles of mastication derived from the somitomeres in branchial arch 1. The sensory neurons in cranial nerve V are derived primarily from neural crest cells that

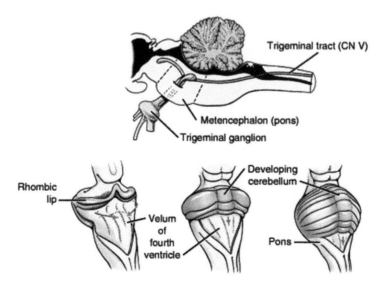

Fig. 11. Development of the metencephalon: surface view and sagittal view of the afferent portion of cranial nerve (CN) V.

form the *trigeminal ganglion*. Most of these neurons are GSA, and their dendritic zones are widely spread over the entire surface of the head and to the mucosa of the components of the respiratory and digestive systems located within the head. A smaller component is composed of general proprioceptive neurons for the muscles and joints in the head region. These sensory neurons greatly outnumber the motor neurons. Therefore, when these sensory axons enter the alar plate region of the metencephalon, they spread out for a short distance rostrally and for a long distance caudally, forming the *spinal tract of the trigeminal nerve* in the pons and medulla. These axons terminate in telodendria at synapses in the alar plate neurons, which form the sensory pontine nucleus of the trigeminal nerve in the pons and the *nucleus of the spinal tract of the trigeminal nerve* in the medulla. This spinal tract and nucleus extend the full length of the medulla and into the first few cervical spinal cord segments where they meet the comparable functional neurons, the substantial gelatinosa (Rexed lamina II), developing in the spinal nerves and spinal cord segment (see **Fig. 11**).

The cerebellum, or dorsal metencephalon, is formed primarily from the proliferation of the germinal epithelial cells of the alar plate, forming the rhombic lip (see **Fig. 11**; **Fig. 12**). This growth dorsolaterally from each side overgrows the roof plate of the fourth ventricle so that the cerebellum forms part of the dorsal boundary of the fourth ventricle in the metencephalon. The ventral metencephalon is the pons. A ventral migration of alar plate mantle layer neurons forms the *pontine nucleus* (see **Fig. 12**). The axons of these neurons cross the midline and course dorsally into the cerebellum. This growth forms the *transverse fibers of the pons*, which demarcate the ventral surface of the pons and the *middle cerebellar peduncle*.

MESENCEPHALON: MIDBRAIN

Symmetric proliferation of the walls of the neural tube in the mesencephalon reduces the size of the neural canal to a narrow tube, the *mesencephalic aqueduct*. This aqueduct is smaller rostrally, where it joins the third ventricle of the diencephalon, and larger caudally, where it is continuous with the fourth ventricle ventral to the rostral medullary velum.

Cranial nerves III (oculomotor) and IV (trochlear) are associated with the midbrain. These contain primarily GSE neurons that innervate extraocular muscles. The cell bodies are in nuclei derived from the basal plate mantle layer. They do not migrate

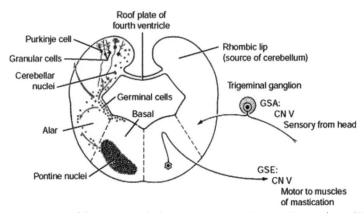

Fig. 12. Development of the metencephalon: transverse section, pontine nucleus. CN, cranial nerve.

but remain adjacent to the median plane ventral to the aqueduct, which is in the same topographic nuclear column as the abducent and hypoglossal GSE nuclei in the medulla (**Fig. 13**). The *parasympathetic nucleus of the oculomotor nerve* is just rostral to the *motor (GSE) nucleus of the oculomotor nerve*. This contains the neuronal cell bodies of the preganglionic parasympathetic axons that innervate the constrictor muscle of the iris. These are derived from the same basal plate mantle layer.

The alar plate proliferates dorsally to form the tectum of the midbrain, which is divided into paired *rostral* and *caudal colliculi,* collectively known as the *corpora quadrigemina*. These colliculi are associated with visual and auditory reflex function, respectively. The *crus cerebri* on the ventral surface of the midbrain results from the caudal growth of caudally projecting axons from telencephalic projection neuronal cell bodies. These axons are continuous from the internal capsule in the diencephalon.

DIENCEPHALON: INTERBRAIN

Rostral to the mesencephalon, the sulcus limitans is no longer evident in the neural tube and the diencephalon and telencephalon are considered to be developments of the alar plate. The symmetric development of the lateral walls of the neural tube in the diencephalon reduces the neural canal to a vertical slit on the median plane, the *third ventricle*. Adhesion of the developing thalamus in the center forms the *interthalamic adhesion* and separates the third ventricle into a small relatively round dorsal component and a larger vertical narrow ventral component. These two portions converge caudally at the mesencephalic aqueduct and rostrally at the level of the *interventricular foramina*, which connect to each telencephalic lateral ventricle (**Fig. 14**). On the dorsal median plane of the diencephalon, there is no proliferation of the neural tube epithelial cells, leaving a single-cell-thick roof plate, where a small *choroid plexus* develops in 2 parallel lines similar to those in the medulla. At the interventricular foramina, each of these is continuous with the choroid plexus that develops in each lateral ventricle (**Fig. 15**).

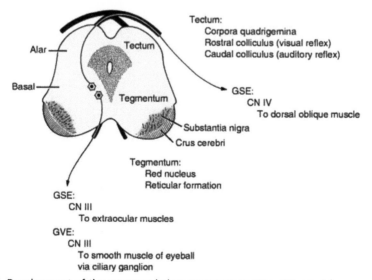

Tectum:
Corpora quadrigemina
Rostral colliculus (visual reflex)
Caudal colliculus (auditory reflex)

Alar
Tectum
Basal
Tegmentum

GSE:
CN IV
To dorsal oblique muscle

Substantia nigra
Crus cerebri

Tegmentum:
Red nucleus
Reticular formation

GSE:
CN III
To extraocular muscles
GVE:
CN III
To smooth muscle of eyeball
via ciliary ganglion

Fig. 13. Development of the mesencephalon: transverse section. CN, cranial nerve.

In the diencephalon, a plethora of nuclei are formed from the mantle layer, which are dispersed diffusely through this brain segment forming a complex of nuclei and neuronal processes.

These nuclei form the *thalamencephalon, hypothalamus, and subthalamus*. The thalamencephalon consists of the *thalamus, metathalamus, and epithalamus*, which comprise those nuclei located dorsal to the ventral portion of the third ventricle. The *hypothalamus* includes the nuclei located on the sides and floor of the ventral portion of the third ventricle. The *subthalamic nuclei* are located ventrolaterally in the

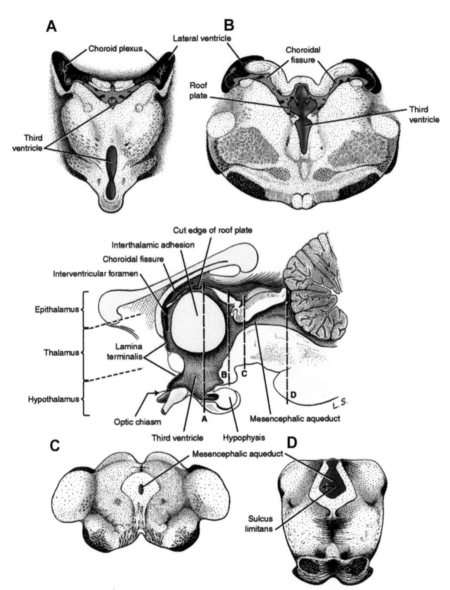

Fig. 14. Relationship of the diencephalon and mesencephalon. (*A*) Transverse section of mid-diencephalon. (*B*) Transverse section of caudal diencephalon. (*C*) Transverse section of rostral mesencephalon. (*D*) Transverse section of caudal mesencephalon.

diencephalon. A ventral outgrowth of the hypothalamus, including an extension of the third ventricle, forms the *neurohypophysis*. The neurohypophysis becomes associated with a dorsal extension of the adjacent oral ectoderm, the *hypophyseal (Rathke) pouch*, to form the *hypophysis (pituitary gland)*. The optic vesicles that initially grew out of the prosencephalon will form the neural layer of the eyes. The axons that grow caudally from the ganglion cell layer of the retina form the prechiasmatic optic tracts (optic nerves), the optic chiasm and the postchiasmatic optic tracts adjacent to the diencephalon. Many of these will terminate in a nuclear area in the thalamus or rostral mesencephalon. The prechiasmatic optic tracts are what has been referred to as the optic nerves, the special somatic afferent neurons of the visual system. By definition, a nerve is a collection of axons outside the CNS that are myelinated by

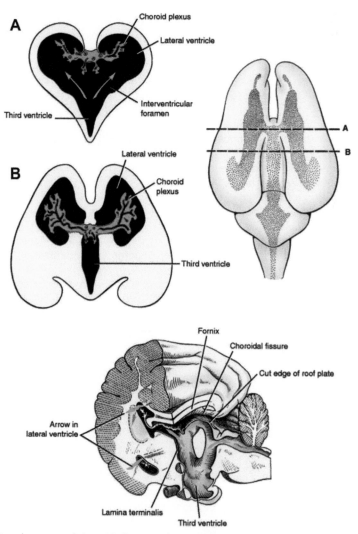

Fig. 15. Development of choroid plexus and ventricular system of diencephalon and telencephalon (*A* and *B* refer to the level of these transverse sections on the drawing of the brain on the *right* side of the figure).

Schwann cells, which arise from the neural crest. Optic nerves are misnamed because they develop as extensions of the prosencephalon and are, therefore, part of the CNS. They form in the optic stalk that extends from the optic cup to the diencephalon. Their axons are myelinated by CNS oligodendroglial cells. Thus, the optic nerve is a tract of the brain that is located rostral to the optic chiasm and should be called the prechiasmatic optic tract. This point is important to remember because the optic nerves are affected by diseases that are specific to the CNS. Therefore, optic neuritis is a form of encephalitis. Conversely, polyneuritis does not affect the optic nerves. Gliomas occur in the prechiasmatic optic tracts.

TELENCEPHALON: CEREBRUM

The rostral boundary of the brainstem is the *lamina terminalis* of the diencephalon. It is the rostral boundary of the third ventricle. The optic chiasm is located at the ventral portion of this lamina, and the *rostral commissure* develops in and remains in this lamina. It is at this level that the telencephalic vesicles grow out of the original single embryonic prosencephalon to form the 2 cerebral hemispheres that comprise the cerebrum. The lamina terminalis is located on the median plane between these two outgrowths. The telencephalic vesicles grow out of the prosencephalon a short distance rostrally and then in a large curve caudally and ventrally. The neural canal in each telencephalon is the *lateral ventricle,* which communicates with the diencephalic third ventricle via the *interventricular foramen* on each side of the lamina terminalis (see **Figs. 15** and **18**).

Each telencephalon forms a *cerebral hemisphere*. The 2 cerebral hemispheres form the single *cerebrum*. The hemispheres are connected by the *corpus callosum*.

At one aspect of the medial wall of the telencephalic vesicle, the neuroepithelial layer of the neural tube does not proliferate and remains a single layer of cells that become ependymal cells comparable with the roof plate of the myelencephalon dorsal to the fourth ventricle and the roof plate of the diencephalon dorsal to the third ventricle. As the rest of the telencephalon proliferates and differentiates, this telencephalic roof plate will be attached to the crus of the *hippocampal fornix* on one side and the *stria terminalis* on the other side. The *choroid plexus* of each lateral ventricle develops in this roof plate as was described for the choroid plexus in the medulla. This choroid plexus is a curved structure similar to the structures that it is attached to, and it protrudes into the lumen of the lateral ventricle. At each *interventricular foramen*, each lateral ventricular choroid plexus is continuous with the choroid plexus of the third ventricle.

An extensive development of projection axons occurs from diencephalic thalamic neurons to the cerebrum and telencephalic neurons to the brainstem. This development gives rise to a thick layer of myelinated processes, white matter, between the diencephalon and telencephalon that is known as the *internal capsule*.

Telencephalic neuronal cell bodies and white matter can be organized as follows.

Cell Bodies

The telencephalic neuronal cell bodies are located in one of two general locations. One is on the external surface of the entire telencephalon, forming the various layers of the *cerebral cortex*. The other is deep to the surface in subcortical *basal nuclei*. These are often incorrectly called basal ganglia. Remember that ganglia are collections of neuronal cell bodies outside the CNS. Such collections inside the CNS are nuclei or cortices. *Cortices* are located superficially, and their neuronal cell bodies are in a continuous arrangement. Examples of basal nuclei are the *caudate nucleus, globus pallidus, putamen, claustrum, and amygdaloid body*. The *cerebral cortex* can be divided into 3 regions based on evolutionary and anatomic features. The *archipallium* (pallium is a synonym for cortex) is the hippocampus, which is an internal gyrus, an area of cerebral cortex that has been rolled into the lateral ventricle and is not visible on the surface of the cerebrum. The *paleopallium* is the olfactory system and is composed of the olfactory bulbs, the peduncles, and the piriform lobe cortex. In animal evolution, these are the most primitive portions of the cerebrum. The *neopallium* is a more recent evolutionary brain development and makes up the surface of all the gyri and sulci of the cerebrum (**Fig. 16**).

Comparative evolutionary studies show the continual development of the neopallium in higher animals, relegating the archipallium and paleopallium to a lesser portion anatomically.

The surface of the amphibian cerebrum is smooth, lacking any gyri. It is composed of the archipallium dorsally, the paleopallium laterally, and the basal nuclei ventrally. In the advanced reptile, the basal nuclei have receded from the ventral surface and have been replaced by the paleopallium on the ventral surface. A small lateral area is neopallium and the dorsal area is archipallium. In mammals, the neopallium has overgrown the other divisions of the cerebral cortex so that the paleopallium is entirely on the ventral surface of the cerebrum, ventral to the *rhinal sulcus*; the archipallium is rolled medially into the lateral ventricle as an internal gyrus, the hippocampus. Continual development of the neopallium in higher mammals has resulted in the characteristic gyri and sulci observed over most of the exposed surface of the cerebrum. The rhinal sulcus separates the neopallium from the paleopallium. This separation is characteristic of all of the domestic animal species; but most laboratory rodents and all birds have no gyri because in these animals the neopallium is unfolded, so the cerebrum has a smooth surface. Although at birth a few gyri and sulci are present in the puppy brain, they increase remarkably during the first 3 to 6 weeks of life.

Axons

The axons of telencephalic neurons form 3 groups of processes based on their destinations. The *association axons* course between cortical areas within one cerebral hemisphere. They can be short and course between adjacent gyri or long and traverse the entire cerebral hemisphere, but they never leave that hemisphere. *Projection axons* leave the cerebral hemisphere where their cell bodies are located and enter the

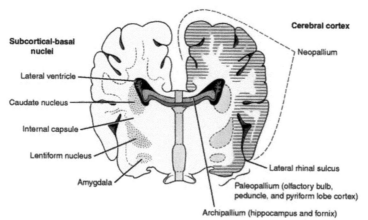

Fig. 16. Development of the neuronal cell bodies in the telencephalon, gray matter.

brainstem via the internal capsule. They terminate in nuclei in various parts of the brainstem, with a few reaching the spinal cord. *Commissural axons* cross from one cerebrum to the other (**Fig. 17**). All of these axons are intermixed in the white matter of each gyrus, which is the *corona radiata,* and in the *centrum semiovale,* which is the mass of white matter in the center of the hemisphere dorsal to the lateral ventricle. The semioval appearance of this structure can be appreciated only in a dorsal plane section of the cerebral hemisphere.

There are 3 groups of commissural axons, all of which initially develop in the lamina terminalis (**Fig. 18**). The *rostral commissure* is located ventrally in the lamina terminalis and courses primarily between paleopallial structures and basal nuclei (the amygdaloid body) on each side. This commissure remains at this site dorsal to the optic chiasm in the fully developed brain. Another small group of commissural axons courses between the archipallium (hippocampus) of each side. This *hippocampal commissure* migrated caudodorsally as the telencephalon developed to reach a position dorsal to the caudal aspect of the diencephalon.

The largest group of commissural axons forms the *corpus callosum,* which also expands dorsally and caudally as the cerebrum develops so that it is positioned between the other two commissures. The corpus callosum serves primarily to connect the neopallial areas of each cerebral hemisphere. It begins in the lamina terminalis; as the telencephalic vesicle expands, the corpus callosum enlarges and extends caudally, dorsal to the diencephalon. Near the median plane it is located between the neopallial cingulate gyrus, dorsally, and the archipallium hippocampus and body of the fornix, ventrally. Laterally in each cerebral hemisphere, the corpus callosum forms the roof of the lateral ventricle. The *septum pellucidum* develops dorsally in the lamina terminalis between the genu of the corpus callosum and the rostral body of the fornix (see **Fig. 18**).

In the telencephalon, the neural tube germinal layer ultimately is replaced by the ependyma of the lateral ventricle. Except for the area of the basal nuclei, the mantle and marginal layers reverse their positions. This reversal is the result of the migration of the newly formed primitive neurons to the surface of the neural tube to form the cerebral cortex, where their axons grow centrally, forming the white matter on the inside of the gray matter. Radial astrocytes participate in this migration by guiding the

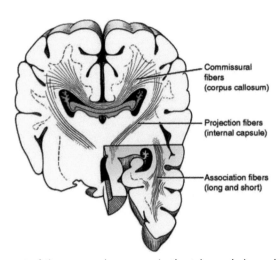

Commissural fibers (corpus callosum)

Projection fibers (internal capsule)

Association fibers (long and short)

Fig. 17. Development of the neuronal processes in the telencephalon, white matter.

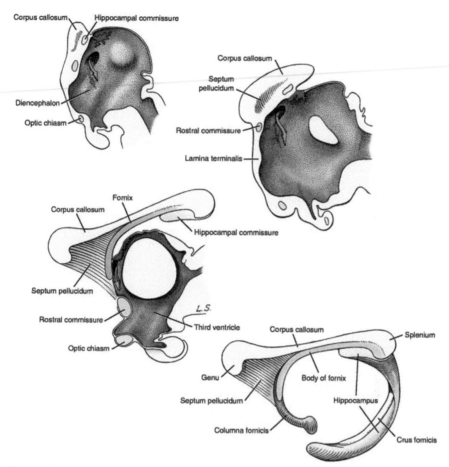

Fig. 18. Development of telencephalic commissural pathways.

neurons to the surface of the neural tube. Ultimately, 6 layers of neurons will populate the cortex and are numbered from superficial (layer I) to deep (layer VI). The first neurons to migrate to the developing cerebral cortex will form layer VI. As more neurons arrive, they pass by those already there to form the rest of the layers in a reverse sequence. Thus, the last to arrive form layer I. The basal nuclei are formed by neurons that migrate only a short distance from the mantle layer into the developing white matter so that they remain in a subcortical position. Remnants of the telencephalic germinal layer persist throughout the life of the animal, forming the subependymal layer, which consists of a variably sized population of small cells that are thought to function as stem cells and serve as a continuous source of glia and neurons throughout the life of the animal. Postnatal neurogenesis is now a well-recognized event, especially in the olfactory system and the hippocampus. This subependymal subventricular layer is thought to be the source of some of the glial neoplasms that arise in the brain and is, therefore, an important region of interest for these types of tumors.

The development of the choroid plexuses of the lateral, third, and fourth ventricles is similar, but the adult morphology varies. The choroid plexuses of the lateral and third ventricle are small and form a thin, undulating veil that projects into the ventricle. The fourth ventricle choroid plexus is more robust and lobulated, especially where it projects through the lateral apertures.

FURTHER READINGS

Bassuk AG, Kibar Z. Genetic basis of neural tube defects. Semin Pediatr Neurol 2009; 16(3):101–10.

Bier E, De Robertis EM. BMP gradients: a paradigm for morphogen-mediated developmental patterning. Science 2015;348(6242):aaa5838.

Butts T, Green MJ, Wingate RJ. Development of the cerebellum: simple steps to make a 'little brain'. Development 2014;141(21):4031–41.

Colas JF, Schoenwolf GC. Towards a cellular and molecular understanding of neurulation. Dev Dyn 2001;221(2):117–45.

Copp AJ, Greene ND. Neural tube defects–disorders of neurulation and related embryonic processes. Wiley Interdiscip Rev Dev Biol 2013;2(2):213–27.

Copp AJ. Neurulation in the cranial region–normal and abnormal. J Anat 2005;207(5): 623–35.

de Lahunta A, Glass E, Kent M. Development of the nervous system: malformations. In: de Lahunta A, Glass EN, Kent M, editors. Veterinary neuroanatomy and clinical neurology. 4th edition. St Louis (MO): Elsevier Saunders; 2015. p. 45–77.

Jiang X, Nardelli J. Cellular and molecular introduction to brain development. Neurobiol Dis 2015. [Epub ahead of print].

Ladhr R, Schoewolf GC. Making a neural tube: neural induction and neurulation. In: Jacobson M, Rao MS, editors. Developmental neurobiology. 4th edition. New York: Kluwer Academic/Plenum; 2005. p. 1–20.

Noden DM, de Lahunta A. Central nervous system and eye. In: Noden DM, de Lahunta A, editors. The embryology of domestic animals: developmental mechanisms and malformations. Baltimore (MD): Williams & Wilkins; 1985. p. 92–119.

Patten I, Placzek M. The role of Sonic hedgehog in neural tube patterning. Cell Mol Life Sci 2000;57(12):1695–708.

Rowitch DH, Kriegstein AR. Developmental genetics of vertebrate glial-cell specification. Nature 2010;468(7321):214–22.

Schoenwolf GC, Smith JL. Mechanisms of neurulation: traditional viewpoint and recent advances. Development 1990;109(2):243–70.

ten Donkelaar HJ, Yamada S, Shiota K, et al. Overview of the development of the human brain and spinal cord. In: ten Donkelaar HJ, Lammens M, Hori A, editors. Clinical neuroembryology: development and developmental disorders of the human central nervous system. 2nd edition. New York: Springer-Heidelberg; 2014. p. 1–52.

Congenital Hydrocephalus

Chelsie M. Estey, MSc, DVM

KEYWORDS

- Hydrocephalus • Brain • Cerebrospinal fluid • Ventricular system
- Ventriculoperitoneal shunt

KEY POINTS

- There are several types of hydrocephalus, which are characterized based on the location of the cerebrospinal fluid (CSF) accumulation.
- Physical features of animals with congenital hydrocephalus may include a dome-shaped skull, persistent fontanelle, and bilateral ventrolateral strabismus.
- Medical therapy involves decreasing the production of CSF.
- The most common surgical treatment is placement of a ventriculoperitoneal shunt.
- Postoperative complications may include infection, blockage, drainage abnormalities, and mechanical failure.

INTRODUCTION

A current definition of hydrocephalus is an active distension of the ventricular system of the brain that results from inadequate movement of cerebrospinal fluid (CSF) from the point of production within the ventricles to its point of absorption.[1] Congenital hydrocephalus typically occurs because of an interruption of CSF flow or defective CSF absorption; hydrocephalus is rarely caused by an increase in CSF production. CSF is formed primarily by the choroid plexus in the lateral, third, and fourth ventricles at a rate of 0.047 mL/min in dogs and 0.017 mL/min in cats.[2] Additional CSF is secreted by the ependymal lining, the external pial-glial membrane on the surface of the brain, and by the blood vessels in the pia-arachnoid.[3,4] Production of CSF is independent of CSF hydrostatic pressure and occurs at a constant rate; however, it depends on osmotic pressure. Normal CSF flow begins in the lateral ventricles and travels through the interventricular foramen to the third ventricle, and from this point it enters the mesencephalic aqueduct to emerge in the fourth ventricle (**Fig. 1**). From the fourth ventricle, CSF exits via the lateral apertures to enter the subarachnoid space. Movement of CSF through the ventricular system is caused by pumping of blood in the choroid plexus. The bulk of CSF absorption takes place at the arachnoid villi and to a lesser degree via venous and lymphatic drainage around spinal and

The author has nothing to disclose.
Upstate Veterinary Specialties, 152 Sparrowbush Road, Latham, NY 12110, USA
E-mail address: cestey@uvsonline.com

Vet Clin Small Anim 46 (2016) 217–229
http://dx.doi.org/10.1016/j.cvsm.2015.10.003
0195-5616/16/$ – see front matter © 2016 Elsevier Inc. All rights reserved.

vetsmall.theclinics.com

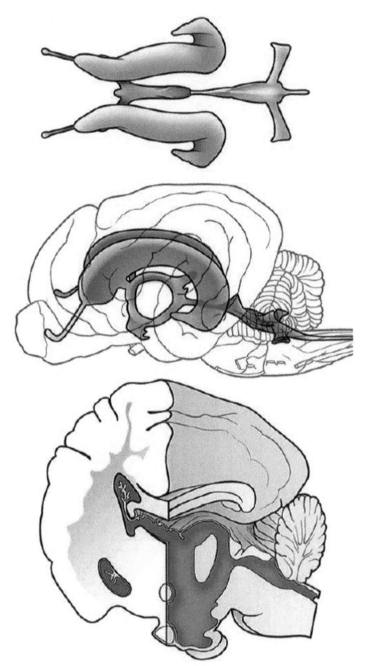

Fig. 1. The normal ventricular anatomy of the canine brain. (*From* Dewey CW, Marino DJ. Congenital brain malformations. In: Tobias KM, Johnston SA, editors. Veterinary surgery, small animal. Philadelphia: Elsevier; 2012. p. 518; with permission.)

cranial nerves. The arachnoid villi are projections of subarachnoid space into the lumen of the venous sinus. The section of the villus that is within the sinus acts as a valve that allows CSF to flow into the lumen of the venous sinus when CSF pressure is higher than venous pressure but collapses when venous pressure is higher, preventing blood from entering the subarachnoid space.[4,5]

TYPES OF HYDROCEPHALUS

Hydrocephalus can be divided into congenital and acquired. There are various types of hydrocephalus, which are characterized based on the location of the CSF accumulation.

- Internal hydrocephalus is the accumulation of CSF within the ventricular system.
- External hydrocephalus is the accumulation of CSF within the subarachnoid space.
- Communicating hydrocephalus is when the CSF in the ventricular system communicates with the subarachnoid space, resulting typically from an obstruction beyond the fourth ventricle.
- An obstructive (or noncommunicating) hydrocephalus is ventricular dilation resulting from a lesion causing obstruction of CSF flow before entering the subarachnoid space.
- A compensatory hydrocephalus can result from loss of central nervous system parenchyma, whereby there is an increase in CSF volume that occupies the space formerly taken up by the lost parenchyma.

PATIENT EVALUATION OVERVIEW

Dogs and cats with congenital hydrocephalus may have signs from birth; however, more commonly signs become apparent in the first few months of life. The rate of clinical progression of congenital hydrocephalus is variable, and some animals may not develop clinical signs of encephalopathy until adulthood. Congenital hydrocephalus is overrepresented in toy breed dogs. Breeds found to be at a higher risk include the Maltese, Yorkshire terrier, English bulldog, Chihuahua, Lhasa apso, Pomeranian, toy poodle, cairn terrier, Boston terrier, pug dog, and Pekingese.[6] The most commonly reported malformation is a stenotic mesencephalic aqueduct, which is often seen with a malformation of the mesencephalon affecting the rostral colliculi and rarely the caudal colliculi.[5] Another potential mechanism is the hydrodynamic theory, which proposes that hydrocephalus develops on account of decreased intracranial compliance, resulting in increased capillary pulse pressure. A pulsatile pressure gradient develops that is directed from the cerebral tissue toward the lateral ventricles. The rebound pressure from the pulsatile gradient, along with the hyperdynamic CSF flow in the mesencephalic aqueduct, results in enlargement of the ventricular system. This enlargement results in congenital hydrocephalus that can develop in the face of normal intracranial pressure.[7] Often a specific cause for the hydrocephalus is not obvious at the time of initial evaluation.

PHYSICAL EXAMINATION FINDINGS

Common physical characteristics of hydrocephalic patients include a large, dome-shaped head, fontanelles or larger calvarial defects, and bilateral ventrolateral strabismus (sun-setting of the eyes) (**Fig. 2**). The strabismus may be the result of either orbital skull malformations or vestibular dysfunction. Dogs and cats with congenital hydrocephalus often show evidence of developmental delay and are smaller than

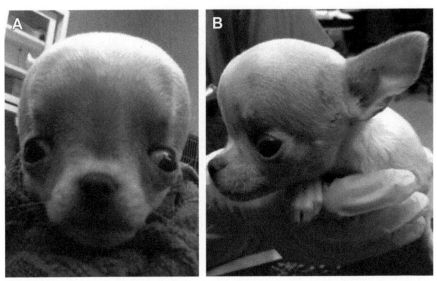

Fig. 2. A frontal (*A*) and lateral (*B*) view of a Chihuahua with congenital hydrocephalus demonstrating an enlarged dome-shaped skull and ventrolateral strabismus.

normal. Clinical signs of neurologic dysfunction usually reflect a forebrain disorder and may include obtundation, behavioral abnormalities, difficulty with training, decreased vision or blindness, circling, pacing, and seizure activity. Concurrent congenital abnormalities of the brain (eg, intracranial arachnoid cyst, Dandy-Walker syndrome, Chiari-like malformation) may also occur in hydrocephalic dogs. Progressive neurologic dysfunction over weeks to months is often a reason for pursuit of medical and/or surgical intervention.

DIAGNOSIS

Diagnosis of congenital hydrocephalus is based on a combination of characteristic clinical features, imaging of the brain to demonstrate ventriculomegaly, and the absence of other causes of encephalopathy. It is important to note that the terms *ventriculomegaly* and *hydrocephalus* are not synonymous. Although enlarged ventricles are a feature of hydrocephalus, not all animals with ventriculomegaly have hydrocephalus. Asymmetric and symmetric enlargement of the lateral ventricles can be seen in neurologically normal animals. In one study looking at normal beagle-type dogs, enlargement of one or both ventricles was seen in 46.7% of the dogs.[8] In another study, the prevalence of asymmetry of the lateral ventricles in a group of 100 neurologically normal dogs was 38%.[9] It is important to use clinical signs and to identify other features on imaging that can help support this diagnosis, such as periventricular hyperintensities on MRI, a site of obstruction, and ventricular enlargement that cannot be entirely attributed to cortical atrophy, to name a few.

IMAGING MODALITIES
Ultrasound

If a dog presents with a persistent fontanelle, then ultrasound may be a safe, minimally invasive modality to image the ventricles. The lateral ventricles would appear enlarged and filled with anechoic fluid and lined by a thin wall. The primary benefit is this can often be done with no sedation. More advanced imaging techniques should be performed following ultrasound evaluation if medical or surgical treatments are to be pursued.

Computed Tomography Scan

Computed tomography (CT) allows visualization of the entire ventricular system. It may be possible to identify a site of obstruction or the morphology of the ventricular system may suggest the location of an obstruction. This modality would also allow visualization of acute hemorrhage. CT can also be used postoperatively to confirm shunt placement (**Fig. 3**).

MRI Scan

MRI will allow for the best resolution and detailed evaluation of the brain parenchyma (**Fig. 4**). Periventricular hyperintensities in the white matter can be seen and often indicate interstitial edema (**Fig. 5**). MRI will also be more useful for identifying concurrent abnormalities (eg, Chiari-like malformation).

MEDICAL TREATMENT

Medical management of hydrocephalus is directed at decreasing the production of CSF. This treatment may be performed in cases when surgery is not an option or in an attempt to stabilize ventricular size and clinical signs until a ventriculoperitoneal shunt can be placed.[10] Antiepileptic drugs may also need to be given if patients are experiencing seizures. Medical therapy may stabilize or improve signs in the short-term, but often it is not successful in the long-term.

Diuretics are used to reduce the production of CSF. Acetazolamide, a carbonic anhydrase inhibitor, has been shown to decrease CSF production by the choroid plexus in both the dog and cat.[11,12] Although acetazolamide can reduce CSF production, this does not always correspond with a reduction in intracranial pressure. In humans with idiopathic normal-pressure hydrocephalus, low-dose acetazolamide has been associated with a reduction in periventricular white matter hyperintensities

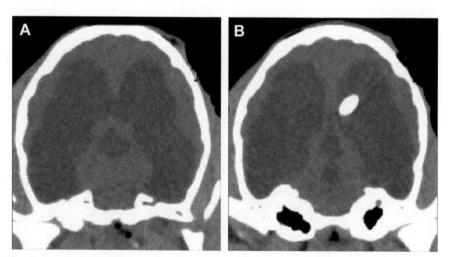

Fig. 3. Preoperative CT scan showing enlarged lateral ventricles in a young dog with congenital hydrocephalus (*A*) and postoperative image showing placement of the ventriculoperitoneal shunt in the lateral ventricle (*B*). (*Courtesy of* Dr Emma Davies, Cornell University Hospital for Animals, Ithaca, NY.)

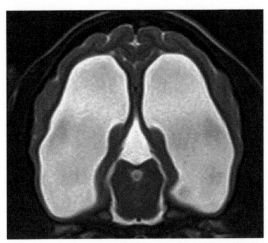

Fig. 4. Transverse T2-weighted image showing dilated lateral ventricles from a hydrocephalic puppy. (*Courtesy of* Dr Emma Davies, Cornell University Hospital for Animals, Ithaca, NY.)

seen on MRI.[13] Furosemide is a loop diuretic that acts mainly by inhibiting sodium reabsorption in the nephron at the thick ascending limb of the loop of Henle.[14] Furosemide has also been shown to decrease CSF production and intracranial pressure in rabbits.[15] Omeprazole is a proton pump inhibitor that has been shown to decrease CSF production and in one study was found to decrease production by 26%.[16,17]

Glucocorticoids are commonly used in patients with hydrocephalus, although there is little published information available regarding their efficacy in these patients. Typically an antiinflammatory dose is used initially; once clinical signs have improved, the medication is tapered to the lowest dose that still controls clinical signs.

Hyperosmolar therapy with agents such as mannitol is occasionally used when there is evidence of intracranial hypertension.[10] Mannitol can reduce intracranial pressure by decreasing blood viscosity, which promotes reflex vasoconstriction; mannitol also produces an osmotic gradient that draws fluid from the brain parenchyma into the

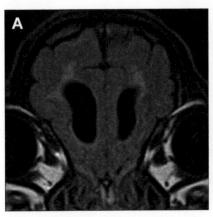
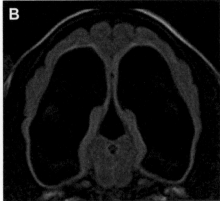

Fig. 5. Transverse fluid attenuated inversion recovery images at the level of the rostral cerebrum (*A*) and mesencephalic aqueduct (*B*) showing dilated lateral ventricles and periventricular hyperintensities. (*Courtesy of* Dr Emma Davies, Cornell University Hospital for Animals, Ithaca, NY.)

vascular space.[18,19] Side effects of mannitol administration may include hypovolemia, electrolyte imbalances, and acute renal failure, so follow-up therapy with isotonic crystalloids may be warranted. Mannitol may result in an initial clinical response but is not suited for long-term therapy, and the response is likely to be transient.[20]

The potential side effects of long-term corticosteroid and/or diuretic therapy need to be considered when deciding about the best course of action for treating congenital hydrocephalus. Electrolyte depletion (particularly potassium) and dehydration are concerns when using diuretics for prolonged time periods, particularly when used in combination with corticosteroids.

Ultrasound-guided ventriculocentesis via the lateral ventricle can be performed in some cases with a persistent fontanelle. This technique can be used to provide temporary relief in clinical patients and also to determine a potential response to placement of a ventriculoperitoneal shunt (**Table 1**).

INDICATIONS FOR SURGERY

There is no clear outline that describes when an animal should have a ventriculoperitoneal shunt placed. Surgical treatment is generally recommended when an animal is showing worsening clinical signs or shows no evidence of improvement or deteriorates when being treated medically. It is important that surgery not be performed in patients with preexisting skin infections at the sites of surgery, systemic infection, or an abdominal infection.[4] Surgical candidates should not have other brain malformations that could be contributing to the neurologic signs that would not get addressed by shunt placement. It is also important to recognize cases that would not benefit from placement of a ventriculoperitoneal shunt, such as those with chronic irreversible changes and those with ventricular enlargement secondary to other causes (eg, cerebral necrosis).[4]

SURGICAL TREATMENT

The use of ventriculoperitoneal shunts is the mainstay for surgical treatment of congenital hydrocephalus. The 4 primary shunt components are a ventricular catheter, a reservoir, a valve, and a distal (peritoneal) catheter. To place a shunt, a burr hole is made in the calvarium lateral to the nuchal crest. The dura mater is incised, and a path for the shunt is made using a needle or stylet gently inserted into the cerebral cortex at the level of the lateral ventricle. The ventricular catheter is placed in the lateral ventricle and is anchored to the skull (**Fig. 6**). The distal portion of the catheter is tunneled subcutaneously and then inserted into the peritoneum via a paralumbar approach. A sufficient amount of additional tubing should be placed in the abdomen to allow for growth of the patients. A catheter can also be placed in the atrium; however, this is technically more challenging, and the jugular vein can be too small for catheter placement in small dogs. It is important to do postoperative imaging to confirm appropriate placement of the shunt (**Figs. 7** and **8**).

Table 1		
A list of medications that have been shown to aid in decreasing CSF production		
Drug	**Class**	**Dosage**
Prednisone	Glucocorticoid	0.25–0.5 mg/kg PO q12h, followed by a taper
Omeprazole	Proton pump inhibitor	1 mg/kg PO q24h
Acetazolamide	Carbonic anhydrase inhibitor	10 mg/kg PO q8h
Furosemide	Loop diuretic	1 mg/kg PO q24h

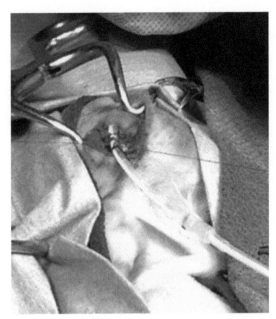

Fig. 6. Intraoperative image of shunt placement in the lateral ventricle for treatment of congenital hydrocephalus. The shunt has been anchored to the calvarium with a Chinese finger trap pattern.

Most of the valves in use are differential pressure valves that will open when the difference in pressure across the valve is greater than the preset opening pressure, which will allow outflow of CSF. When the pressure difference decreases below the set point, the valve closes, stopping movement of CSF.[21,22] Externally programmable valves are also available, which allow the clinician to noninvasively adjust the opening pressure by use of a magnetic device. Depending on the variety, some of the programmable valves can be reset in the MRI machine, whereas others have a locking mechanism in place to prevent this. Most valves are compatible with MRI machines up to 3 T; however, evaluation after imaging and readjustment of the settings may be needed to ensure that correct opening pressure is maintained.[23,24]

SURGICAL COMPLICATIONS

Ventriculoperitoneal shunting is a well-established practice in the treatment of congenital hydrocephalus. Most patients tolerate the surgery and show improvements postoperatively. However, there are several well-known complications that can be seen with this procedure.

Infection

Shunt infections are seen in approximately 8% of cases in people and are typically identified within 2 months of surgery.[21] Treatment of an infection often requires removal of the shunt, culturing the organism, and instituting treatment based on sensitivity results. MRI features of a shunt-associated infection have been outlined in a dog. These features included T2-weighted and fluid-attenuated inversion recovery hyperintensity of the ventricular lining and marked contrast enhancement of the ependymal layer on T1-weighted postcontrast images.[25]

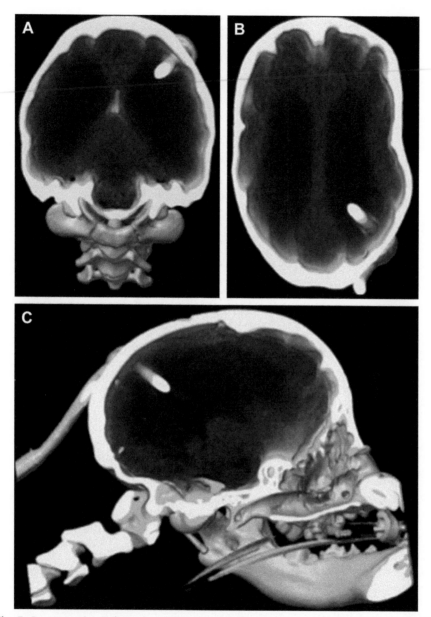

Fig. 7. Postoperative 3-dimensional CT reconstruction images in transverse (*A*), dorsal (*B*), and sagittal (*C*) planes showing shunt placement in the lateral ventricle. (*Courtesy of* Dr Emma Davies, Cornell University Hospital for Animals, Ithaca, NY.)

Blockage

Various components of the shunt can become blocked. Blockage can occur as a result of debris (tissue, hemorrhage, highly cellular CSF) occluding the catheter, obstruction by choroid plexus, the tip of the catheter becoming lodged within or against the brain parenchyma, and the peritoneal portion of the catheter can become occluded or similarly embedded within or against tissue. It is also possible for the

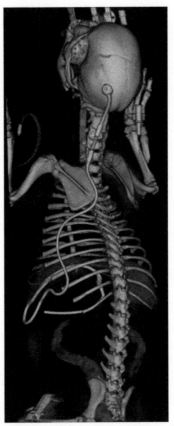

Fig. 8. Postoperative 3-dimensional CT dorsal plane reconstruction image showing place-ment of the ventriculoperitoneal shunt. (*Courtesy of* Dr Emma Davies, Cornell University Hospital for Animals, Ithaca, NY.)

shunt to become kinked, which would prevent adequate drainage. Blockage may require surgical exploration and replacement of the faulty component.

Drainage

It is possible that overdrainage can cause the ventricles to collapse. This collapse can result in CSF that accumulates between the brain and skull and can also cause sub-dural hematoma formation secondary to tearing of the vasculature. In these cases, a valve with a higher opening pressure or a device with a programmable valve may be needed. Underdrainage can result when the catheter system is blocked, becomes disconnected, or is kinked.

Mechanical Failure

Shunt malfunction can be the result of breakage, migration, or disconnection of one or multiple components of the shunt.

PROGNOSIS

Overall the success rate for dogs treated with shunting falls in the range of 72% to 100%.[26–29] In one recent veterinary study evaluating 36 cases of congenital hydrocephalus in dogs and cats, it was found that there was an overall improvement in clinical signs in 72% of the animals. Twenty-two percent of the animals developed post-operative complications, and 36% of the animals died of hydrocephalus-related compli-cations or were euthanized.[27] As in people, this study found that most complications were seen within a few months following surgical intervention. In another study of 14 dogs, ventriculoperitoneal shunting was successful in improving neurologic signs in most dogs, and postoperative complications were seen in 29% of the patients; but these complications could be addressed either medically or surgically.[28] In a study of 12 dogs with hydrocephalus that underwent ventriculoperitoneal shunting, all showed signs of neurologic improvement after shunt placement; however, 25% of the dogs were eutha-nized because of a lack of sustained improvement or skull pain. The other animals had sustained improvement, and one did require revision surgery.[29] In a human study look-ing at ventriculoperitoneal shunt placement outcomes in infants, it was found that the risk of shunt failure was higher in infants less than 1 month of age at the time of shunt placement.[30] In another human study of 198 pediatric patients with hydrocephalus, it was found that 8.6% of patients experienced shunt infections and they were more likely to be underweight compared with those without infection. In this study the mean interval between shunt placement and infection was 1.83 ± 1.25 months and coagulase-negative *Staphylococcus* was the most commonly encountered pathogen.[31] In a human study of 333 consecutive ventriculoperitoneal shunts placed in pediatric patients, it was found that 35 shunts (10.5%) were infected and that infection occurred at a median of 1 months after shunt placement.[32] As in the previously mentioned study, the most com-mon causative agent was coagulase-negative *Staphylococcus*. This study also found that an independent risk factor for infection was having surgery before 1 year of age.[32] Similar investigations looking at risk factors have not been performed in veterinary medicine, but it is possible that age could be a risk factor in veterinary patients as well, for similar reasons, such as less developed immune systems, immaturity of the skin bar-rier, and the population of bacterial flora.[30,32]

It is important to have a detailed discussion with the owners regarding the potential complications associated with this surgery and the possible need for a revision sur-gery should these issues be encountered postoperatively. As in human medicine, complications are most commonly seen in the first few months following surgery, so frequent reevaluation is important in the early postoperative period.

Presently, placement of a ventriculoperitoneal shunt in patients with congenital hydrocephalus is still the best treatment option in those animals that are deemed to be appropriate surgical candidates.

REFERENCES

1. Rekate HL. A contemporary definition and classification of hydrocephalus. Semin Pediatr Neurol 2009;16:9–15.
2. deLahunta A. Cerebrospinal fluid and hydrocephalus. In: deLahunta A, editor. Veterinary neuroanatomy and clinical neurology. 2nd edition. Philadelphia: WB Saunders Co; 1983. p. 30–52.
3. Speake T, Whitwell C, Kajita H, et al. Mechanisms of CSF secretion by the choroid plexus. Microsc Res Tech 2001;52:49–59.
4. Thomas WB. Hydrocephalus in dogs and cats. Vet Clin North Am Small Anim Pract 2010;40:143–59.
5. deLahunta A, Glass E, Kent M. Cerebrospinal fluid and hydrocephalus. In: deLahunta A, Glass E, Kent M, editors. Veterinary neuroanatomy and clinical neurology. 4th edition. St Louis (MO): Elsevier Saunders; 2015. p. 78–101.

6. Selby LA, Hayes HM Jr, Becker SV. Epizootiologic features of canine hydrocephalus. Am J Vet Res 1979;40:411–3.
7. Dewey CW, da Costa RC. Practical guide to canine and feline neurology. 3rd edition. Ames (IA): Wiley-Blackwell; 2016. p. 688.
8. Kii S, Uzuka Y, Taura Y, et al. Magnetic resonance imaging of the lateral ventricles in beagle-type dogs. Vet Radiol Ultrasound 1997;38:430–3.
9. Pivetta M, De Risio L, Newton R, et al. Prevalence of lateral ventricle asymmetry in brain MRI studies of neurologically normal dogs and dogs with idiopathic epilepsy. Vet Radiol Ultrasound 2013;54:516–21.
10. Poca MA, Sahuquillo J. Short-term medical management of hydrocephalus. Expert Opin Pharmacother 2005;6:1525–38.
11. Maren TH. Carbonic anhydrase: chemistry, physiology, and inhibition. Physiol Rev 1967;47:595–781.
12. Vogh BP. The relation of choroid plexus carbonic anhydrase activity to cerebrospinal fluid formation: study of three inhibitors in cat with extrapolation to man. J Pharmacol Exp Ther 1980;213:321–31.
13. Alperin N, Oliu CJ, Bagci AM, et al. Low-dose acetazolamide reverses periventricular white matter hyperintensities in iNPH. Neurology 2014;82:1347–51.
14. Eades SK, Christensen ML. The clinical pharmacology of loop diuretics in the pediatric patient. Pediatr Nephrol 1998;12:603–16.
15. Lorenzo AV, Hornig G, Zavala LM, et al. Furosemide lowers intracranial pressure by inhibiting CSF production. Z Kinderchir 1986;41(Suppl 1):10–2.
16. Javaheri S, Corbett WS, Simbartl LA, et al. Different effects of Omeprazole and Sch 28080 on canine cerebrospinal fluid production. Brain Res 1997;754:321–4.
17. Lindvall-Axelsson M, Nilsson C, Owman C, et al. Inhibition of cerebrospinal fluid formation by omeprazole. Exp Neurol 1992;115:394–9.
18. Kukreti V, Mohseni-Bod H, Drake J. Management of raised intracranial pressure in children with traumatic brain injury. J Pediatr Neurosci 2014;9:207–15.
19. Fink ME. Osmotherapy for intracranial hypertension: mannitol versus hypertonic saline. Continuum (Minneap Minn) 2012;18:640–54.
20. Hayden PW, Foltz EL, Shurtleff DB. Effect of on oral osmotic agent on ventricular fluid pressure of hydrocephalic children. Pediatrics 1968;41:955–67.
21. Thompson D. Hydrocephalus. Neurosurgery 2009;27(3):130–4.
22. Corns R, Martin A. Hydrocephalus. Surgery 2012;30:142–8.
23. Lollis SS, Mamourian AC, Vaccaro TJ, et al. Programmable CSF shunt valves: radiographic identification and interpretation. AJNR Am J Neuroradiol 2010;31:1343–6.
24. Lavinio A, Harding S, Van Der Boogaard F, et al. Magnetic field interactions in adjustable hydrocephalus shunts. J Neurosurg Pediatr 2008;2:222–8.
25. Platt SR, McConnell JF, Matiasek L. Imaging diagnosis–ventriculo-peritoneal shunt associated infection in a dog. Vet Radiol Ultrasound 2012;53:80–3.
26. Gage ED. Surgical treatment of canine hydrocephalus. J Am Vet Med Assoc 1970;157:1729–40.
27. Biel M, Kramer M, Forterre F, et al. Outcome of ventriculoperitoneal shunt implantation for treatment of congenital internal hydrocephalus in dogs and cats: 36 cases (2001-2009). J Am Vet Med Assoc 2013;242:948–58.
28. de Stefani A, de Risio L, Platt SR, et al. Surgical technique, postoperative complications and outcome in 14 dogs treated for hydrocephalus by ventriculoperitoneal shunting. Vet Surg 2011;40:183–91.
29. Shihab N, Davies E, Kenny PJ, et al. Treatment of hydrocephalus with ventriculoperitoneal shunting in twelve dogs. Vet Surg 2011;40:477–84.

30. Maruyama H, Nakata Y, Kanazawa A, et al. Ventriculoperitoneal shunt outcomes among infants. Acta Med Okayama 2015;69:87–93.
31. Uche EO, Onyia E, Mezue UC, et al. Determinants and outcomes of ventriculo-peritoneal shunt infections in Enugu, Nigeria. Pediatr Neurosurg 2013;49:75–80.
32. Lee JK, Seok JY, Lee JH, et al. Incidence and risk factors of ventriculoperitoneal shunt infections in children: a study of 333 consecutive shunts in 6 years. J Korean Med Sci 2012;27:1563–8.

Chiari-like Malformation

Catherine A. Loughin, DVM

KEYWORDS

- Chiari-like malformation • Syringomyelia • Occipital hypoplasia
- Foramen magnum decompression

KEY POINTS

- Chiari-like malformation is a condition in which there is a relatively small caudal cranial fossa volume with associated crowding of the brain parenchyma.
- Chiari-like malformation is diagnosed on MRI by identifying cerebellar herniation, cerebellar compression, and attenuation of cerebrospinal fluid, but kinking of the medulla, ventriculomegaly/hydrocephalus, and syringomyelia are also noted in many dogs.
- Some patients respond favorably to medical management; foramen magnum decompression with a durotomy is the surgical treatment of choice in improving or resolving clinical signs in dogs with Chiari-like malformation.

Chiari-like malformation (CLM) is a condition of the craniocervical junction in which there is a mismatch of the structures of the caudal cranial fossa (CCF), often causing the cerebellum to herniate into the foramen magnum.[1–4] Affected dogs have a smaller CCF with relatively more brain parenchyma within the fossa compared to unaffected dogs.[2,3,5–8] This smaller CCF leads to cerebellar compression and herniation through the foramen magnum, kinking of the medulla, and disruption of cerebrospinal fluid (CSF) at this junction.[2,3,5,9,10] This malformation is found most commonly in the Cavalier King Charles spaniel (CKCS), is inherited,[11–14] and is thought to affect as much as 95% of the population.[15] However, CLM has also been diagnosed in the Griffon Bruxellois and many other small breed dogs[13,14,16,17] and is also analogous to Chiari type 1 malformation in humans.[18,19]

PATHOPHYSIOLOGY

Chiari type 1 malformation in people results from hypoplasia of the basioccipital bone and a subsequent decreased volume of the posterior cranial fossa secondarily overcrowding the hindbrain parenchyma and causing herniation of the cerebellum through the foramen magnum.[18,20] Morphologic analyses in CKCS have assessed

The author has nothing to disclose.
Department of Surgery, Canine Chiari Institute, Long Island Veterinary Specialists, 163 South Service Road, Plainview, NY 11803, USA
E-mail address: cloughin@livs.org

Vet Clin Small Anim 46 (2016) 231–242
http://dx.doi.org/10.1016/j.cvsm.2015.10.002   **vetsmall.theclinics.com**
0195-5616/16/$ – see front matter © 2016 Elsevier Inc. All rights reserved.

the CCF.[2,3,5–7,21] When compared with mesaticephalic breeds, CKCS have a shallower CCF and abnormal suboccipital and basioccipital bone.[2] A recent study also showed that CKCS had an 80% probability for closure of the spheno-occipital synchondrosis at 8 months of age, whereas brachycephalic dogs closed at 12 months and mesatice-phalics closed at 16 months, supporting the theory that abnormal skull shape contrib-utes to CKCS predisposition for CLM.[22] CKCSs also have overcrowding as noted in humans, but in comparison to brachycephalics and other small breed dogs, there is no reported difference in CCF volume[5,7] or an association between CCF volume and subsequent syringomyelia (SM).[3,6,23] One study showed that CKCS with SM had increased volume of brain parenchyma compared with CKCS without SM.[6] However, when compared with other dogs, one study found that relative volume of hindbrain pa-renchyma in the CKCS is greater than other small breed dogs and approximately equal to mesaticephalic,[5] but was refuted in another study that showed the CKCS has a rela-tively larger cerebellum than small breed dogs and Labrador retrievers.[4]

SM is a condition in which fluid accumulates within the spinal cord.[24,25] Normally, CSF circulates from the ventricular system to the subarachnoid space. Movement of CSF within the subarachnoid space of the cranial cavity and to the spinal cord is dependent on the cardiac systole and intracranial arterial pulsations. Any obstruc-tion to the normal flow of CSF can lead to the development of SM.[4,6,8] Syrinx forma-tion secondary to CLM is not fully understood, but is thought to be multifactorial. These factors are structural abnormalities coupled with changes in CSF and blood flow.

Craniospinal compliance is the ability of cranial and spinal compartments to accom-modate changes in the parenchymal, blood, or CSF volumes.[26] Compliance can be affected by changes in the skull, CSF volume or flow, vasculature and blood flow, and space-occupying lesions. In CLM, there are 2 potential outcomes of reduced compliance. Obstruction to CSF flow at the foramen magnum could lead to retention of the CSF in the skull and can be manifested as ventriculomegaly.[6,17,27,28] Reduced compliance might affect the shift of pressure between blood and CSF and could lead to the turbulent CSF flow at the foramen magnum leading to SM.[28–31]

Two other findings add to the theories of syrinx formation. First, syrinx fluid has been documented to be at a higher pressure than CSF in the subarachnoid space.[32] Second, CSF communicates with the subarachnoid space via perivascular spaces.[33,34] It has been proposed that SM results from a delay in the peak CSF pulse pressure that arrives at the arteries when they are small, the perivascular spaces are larger, and resistance to CSF is at its lowest, creating a 1-way valve in the perivascular spaces for pulsatile CSF flow against the normal pressure gradient.[35]

CLINICAL SIGNS

Neuropathic pain and associated abnormal sensations represent the most common clinical sign in dogs with CLM. Pain can be manifested as allodynia (pain from nonnox-ious stimuli), hyperesthesia sensitivity to touch and temperature, and paresthesia (spontaneous prickly sensation).[27,36] These sensations can be detected on physical examination and can also be manifested as "phantom scratching" or "air-guitar" (scratching without making contact with the skin).[27,37,38] Other manifestations of sen-soral abnormalities include facial rubbing on the floor or furniture, exercise intolerance, and inability to tolerate a neck collar.[10,38–40]

Dogs with SM exhibit signs of pain secondary to disruption to the fibers of the dor-sal horn laminae.[37,38,41,42] Asymmetric syrinxes have been shown to cause neuro-pathic pain, and specifically in CKCS, syrinx width was the strongest predictor of pain, scratching, and scoliosis.[41,42] In a group of Griffon Bruxellois, it was noted that the neurologic deficits, not pain, were significantly associated with larger syrinxes, and syrinx size increased with age.[43] Histopathologically, dogs with SM have degenerative changes associated with neuronal necrosis and Wallerian degeneration, and disruption of ependymal integrity followed by angiogenesis and fibrous tissue proliferation around blood vessels.[41] This type of syrinx damage to the gray matter is associated with clinical signs.

Other neurologic signs noted in dogs with CLM are facial nerve deficits, seizures, vestibular syndrome, ataxia, menace deficit, proprioceptive deficits, head tremor, temporal muscle atrophy, and multifocal central nervous signs.[10,36–38,44–46] Scoliosis is suspected to be a consequence of SM. It can result from damage to lower motor neurons of the ventral gray matter of the spinal cord, resulting in paraspinal muscle atrophy and asymmetric muscle tone.[36,38,47,48] There has been one report of dysphagia in a CKCS,[49] which is a clinical sign that has been noted in people with Chiari.[50–54]

Dogs of all ages may present with CLM, but most commonly signs develop in younger dogs. Many studies list a mean age around 2 to 4 years with a range from a few months to older than 10 years of age.[10,45,46,55] There is also no reported sex predisposition for CLM.[1,23,46]

DIAGNOSIS

MRI is the modality of choice in the diagnosis of CLM. CLM is diagnosed by identifying the following abnormalities: caudal cerebellar herniation, caudal cerebellar compression from occipital dysplasia, and attenuation of CSF, but kinking of the medulla, ventriculomegaly/hydrocephalus, and SM are also noted in many dogs with CLM.[3,10,44] Midsagittal (**Fig. 1**) and axial images are evaluated, and measurements can be performed to assess for linear and volume changes associated with the brain and cervical regions.[2,3,9] These same images can also be assessed for other neurologic conditions that may cause similar signs or occur concurrently, such as hydrocephalus, intracranial cysts, intervertebral disc disease, and vertebral column malformations. In a large study involving 274 dogs being evaluated for CLM, the

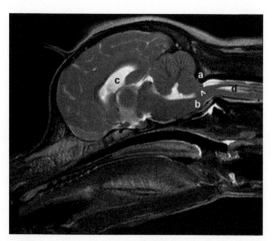

Fig. 1. Sagittal T2-weighted MRI of a dog with CLM and SM. Cerebellar compression and herniation (*a*), medullary kinking (*b*), ventriculomegaly (*c*), syrinx (*d*), and attenuation of CSF (*arrowhead*).

investigators found that atlanto-occipital overlap was diagnosed in 76 (27.7%) dogs and may be an important differential in the diagnosis of CLM.[9] Primary secretory otitis media (PSOM) is seen as hyperintensity in the bulla on MRI T2-weighted axial images and is very common in CKCS with CLM.[56–58] Clinical signs for PSOM can be similar to CLM, so careful assessment of the patient and the MRI is necessary for an accurate diagnosis.

SM appears as a linear hyperintensity on sagittal T2-weighted images of the spinal cord. The width and dorsal horn involvement can be assessed on axial T2-weighted images (**Fig. 2**). SM can be seen over one vertebra or several (**Fig. 3**). One study revealed C1-4 and T-L2 are the most common areas for SM to be noted[59]; therefore, imaging of the entire spine is recommended.

Phase-contrast MRI, or cine MRI, has improved the assessment of CSF flow through the craniocervical junction. This modality combines flow-dependent contrast with cardiac gating (MRI sequence acquired by electrocardiogram recordings during image acquisition) to produce images throughout the cardiac cycle. This technique has been used to assess CSF flow in CKCS and has shown that flow obstruction at the foramen magnum causes turbulent flow that is associated with SM presence and severity.[24,29] This modality may be used to monitor clinical progression and also assess for resolution after decompressive surgery.[24,29,60]

Computed tomography (CT) can also be used in the assessment of CLM. Helical CT scanners allow for image reconstruction and analysis for linear measurements and volume calculations. Morphometric analysis of the cranial cavity and CCF in normal dogs have suggested CT may be useful in the assessment of dogs with suspect CLM,[21,23] whereas a study comparing CT and MRI concluded that both modalities are capable of detecting cerebellar herniation and determining cerebellar herniation length.[61]

Ultrasound has been used to assess the craniocervical junction to identify cerebellar herniation and compression and medullary kink, but is limited in assessment for SM due to bone overlay.[23,62] Evaluation of CSF in dogs with CLM or SM had higher nucleated cell counts, increased protein levels, and an increase in neutrophils and lymphocytes, but it can be normal as well.[37,44,63–65]

TREATMENT

Medical and surgical treatment options are available for CLM. Medical treatment is commonly instituted for pain relief and reduction of CSF production, but does not prevent disease progression and only provides temporary relief from clinical signs in many dogs.[46,66,67] In a study of CKCS medically managed for CLM and SM over 39 months, the investigators found that 75% of the cases had progression of

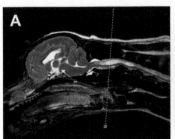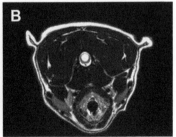

Fig. 2. (*A*) Sagittal T2-weighted MRI of a dog with CLM and SM (*dashed line* marks the location of the axial figure on the sagittal image). (*B*) Corresponding axial image.

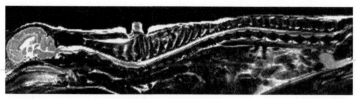

Fig. 3. A full-body sagittal T2-weighted MRI of a dog with a syrinx that extends to the lumbar spine.

clinical signs.[39] In contrast, 3 studies evaluating surgical treatment of CLM with greater than 1 year follow-up showed that 80% to 81% of the dogs had clinical improvement.[44,45,55] Given these observations, there are some dogs that do not need surgery, but many more that will progress clinically without surgical intervention.

Pain secondary to CLM has been typically managed with nonsteroidal anti-inflammatory drugs (NSAIDs), anticonvulsants, corticosteroids, and opioids. Multimodal medical management more frequently controls clinical signs over a single drug class.[68] Cyclo-oxygenase inhibition used by NSAIDs has been shown to help alleviate neuropathic pain.[69] Coxibs, deracoxib (Deramax) and fibrocoxib (Previcox), are lipophilic and reach significant CSF concentrations that may provide analgesia via a central action.[70,71] Two anticonvulsants have been reported to be effective for neuropathic pain, gabapentin (Neurontin) and pregabalin (Lyrica). Gabapentin is thought to prevent the release of glutamate at the dorsal horn by interaction with the $\alpha 2\delta$ subunit of the voltage-gated calcium channels, and pregabalin is thought to also work at voltage-gated calcium channels, resulting in a decrease in glutamate and substance P.[27,72–74] Corticosteroids not only have an anti-inflammatory effect, they also have an effect on sympathetically mediated pain by decreased substance P expression.[27,66,75] Tramadol (Ultram) is a synthetic opioid that interacts with μ-opioid receptors and has effects on serotonin and norepinephrine reuptake.[76] A tricyclic antidepressant, amitryptilline (Elavil), has been prescribed for dogs with CLM because it has been prescribed for neuropathic pain in humans, but it is unknown if it is effective for neuropathic pain in dogs.[27,77]

Injectable pain management is typically used in the perioperative period. Ketamine (Ketalar), a N-methyl-D-aspartate antagonist, is a proven drug for neuropathic pain, as well as the sodium channel blocker, lidocaine.[27,77,78] Injectable opioids provide perioperative analgesia as well.

Many owners ask for nonpharmaceutical options for pain management. Acupuncture significantly affects the autonomic nervous system and has been used for neuropathic pain in dogs with CLM.[27,45] Low-level laser therapy is becoming more popular in veterinary medicine to decrease pain. A study in humans with neck pain has shown some promising results for pain relief,[79] but studies still need to be performed to assess its value in dogs with CLM.

Medical management also includes drugs that reduce CSF production. Omeprazole (Prilosec), a proton pump inhibitor, may be helpful in decreasing CSF pulse pressure.[80,81] Acetazolamide (Diamox) and methazolamide (Nepatazane), carbonic anhydrase inhibitors, also decrease CSF flow.[82–84] Furosemide (Lasix) decreases intracranial pressure by diuresis and reduced blood volume,[85,86] but it may not have the effect on CSF pressure that is desired.[87] Corticosteroids, such as prednisone, may also decrease CSF pressure.[88]

Surgical decompression of the foramen magnum is the treatment of choice for humans with Chiari type 1 malformation[89–92] and is also the surgical treatment used by many veterinary neurosurgeons. Foramen magnum decompression (FMD) is a suboccipital craniotomy with a dorsal laminectomy of the first cervical vertebra (**Fig. 4**).[44,46,55,67] This FMD is followed by a durotomy over the atlanto-occipital and atlantoaxial regions to re-establish CSF flow through the region.[44,55,67] Surgery offers a long-term treatment option for dogs with progressive clinical signs or dogs that have failed medical management. FMD has been able to improve or resolve clinical signs in approximately 80% of dogs.[44,55] Early surgical intervention has also been recommended.[44,67] Most postoperative improvement is in the form of reduced pain and neurologic signs, but many dogs experience residual scratching that can be managed with medication long term.[45]

Despite the success of FMD in controlling symptoms, recurrence of clinical signs has been noted in 25% to 47% of dogs.[44,55] The reason for the recurrence or worsening of symptoms is thought to be related to compressive scar tissue formation, in most cases. Reconstruction of the caudal occipital region after FMD, also known as a cranioplasty (**Fig. 5**), has lessened the incidence of postoperative scar tissue formation in humans.[93–95] Many cranioplasties performed in people are formulated from autologous bone grafts, but one made from titanium mesh has been used in humans and dogs.[45,95] In one canine study in which a titanium mesh/polymethylmethacrylate plate cranioplasty was performed following FMD, none of the dogs required a second surgery for scar tissue formation during the study period.[45] A larger, long-term study is currently being completed to further investigate improvement/resolution of clinical signs as well as the rate of postoperative scar tissue formation with cranioplasty (Loughin 2015, unpublished).

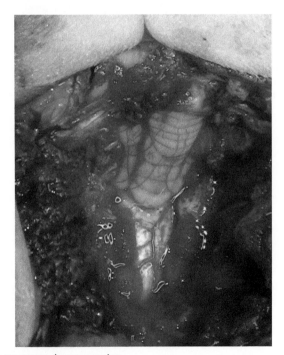

Fig. 4. Foramen magnum decompression.

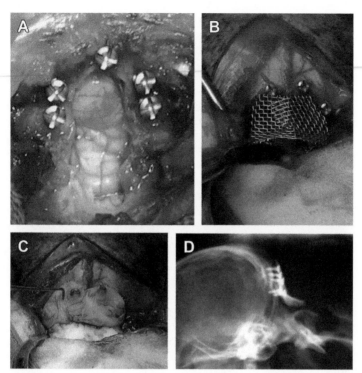

Fig. 5. (*A*) Placement of the titanium screws for an FMD with cranioplasty. (*B*) Placement of the titanium mesh. (*C*) Cranioplasty in place with polymethylmethacrylate. (*D*) Postoperative lateral radiograph of the cranioplasty implants in place over the occiput/C1.

SUMMARY

CLM is an abnormality of the craniocervical junction that most commonly affects CKCS, but may be diagnosed in many other small breed dogs. Pain and scratching are the most common clinical signs, but other symptoms attributable to the central nervous system have been reported. Advanced imaging is necessary for diagnosis, and MRI is the diagnostic of choice to fully evaluate the craniocervical junction for structural abnormalities as well as the entire spinal cord for SM. Medical management can provide some dogs with sustainable pain relief, but surgical decompression has been shown to improve clinical signs in approximately 80% of dogs.

REFERENCES

1. Cappello R, Rusbridge C. Report from the chiari-like malformation and syringomyelia working group round table. Vet Surg 2007;36:509–12.
2. Carrera I, Dennis R, Mellor DJ, et al. Use of magnetic resonance imaging for morphometric analysis of the caudal cranial fossa in Cavalier King Charles Spaniels. Am J Vet Res 2009;70:340–5.
3. Cerda-Gonzalez S, Olby NJ, McCullough S, et al. Morphology of the caudal fossa in Cavalier King Charles Spaniels. Vet Radiol Ultrasound 2009;50:37–46.
4. Shaw TA, McGonnell IM, Driver CJ, et al. Caudal cranial fossa partitioning in Cavalier King Charles spaniels. Vet Rec 2013;172:341.

5. Cross HR, Cappello R, Rusbridge C. Comparison of cerebral cranium volumes between cavalier King Charles spaniels with Chiari-like malformation, small breed dogs and Labradors. J Small Anim Pract 2009;50:399–405.

6. Driver CJ, Rusbridge C, Cross HR, et al. Relationship of brain parenchyma within the caudal cranial fossa and ventricle size to syringomyelia in cavalier King Charles spaniels. J Small Anim Pract 2010;51:382–6.

7. Schmidt MJ, Biel M, Klumpp S, et al. Evaluation of the volumes of cranial cavities in Cavalier King Charles Spaniels with Chiari-like malformation and other brachyce-phalic dogs as measured via computed tomography. Am J Vet Res 2009;70:508–12.

8. Driver CJ, Rusbridge C, McGonnell IM, et al. Morphometric assessment of cranial volumes in age-matched Cavalier King Charles spaniels with and without syringo-myelia. Vet Rec 2010;167:978–9.

9. Marino DJ, Loughin CA, Dewey CW, et al. Morphometric features of the craniocer-vical junction region in dogs with suspected Chiari-like malformation determined by combined use of magnetic resonance imaging and computed tomography. Am J Vet Res 2012;73:105–11.

10. Lu D, Lamb CR, Pfeiffer DU, et al. Neurological signs and results of magnetic resonance imaging in 40 cavalier King Charles spaniels with Chiari type 1-like malformations. Vet Rec 2003;153:260–3.

11. Lewis T, Rusbridge C, Knowler P, et al. Heritability of syringomyelia in Cavalier King Charles spaniels. Vet J 2010;183:345–7.

12. Rusbridge C, Knowler P, Rouleau GA, et al. Inherited occipital hypoplasia/syrin-gomyelia in the cavalier King Charles spaniel: experiences in setting up a world-wide DNA collection. J Hered 2005;96:745–9.

13. Rusbridge C, Knowler SP. Hereditary aspects of occipital bone hypoplasia and syringomyelia (Chiari type I malformation) in Cavalier King Charles spaniels. Vet Rec 2003;153:107–12.

14. Rusbridge C, Knowler SP. Inheritance of occipital bone hypoplasia (Chiari type I malformation) in Cavalier King Charles Spaniels. J Vet Intern Med 2004;18:673–8.

15. Dewey CRC. Treatment of canine Chiari-like malformation and syringomyelia. In: Bongura J, Twedt DC, editors. Kirk's current veterinary therapy. St Louis (MO): Saunders Elsevier; 2008. p. 1102–7.

16. Rusbridge C. Neurological diseases of the Cavalier King Charles spaniel. J Small Anim Pract 2005;46:265–72.

17. Rusbridge C, Knowler SP, Pieterse L, et al. Chiari-like malformation in the Griffon Bruxellois. J Small Anim Pract 2009;50:386–93.

18. Milhorat TH, Nishikawa M, Kula RW, et al. Mechanisms of cerebellar tonsil herni-ation in patients with Chiari malformations as guide to clinical management. Acta Neurochir (Wien) 2010;152:1117–27.

19. Fernandez AA, Guerrero AI, Martinez MI, et al. Malformations of the craniocervi-cal junction (Chiari type I and syringomyelia: classification, diagnosis and treat-ment). BMC Musculoskelet Disord 2009;10(Suppl 1):S1.

20. Milhorat TH, Chou MW, Trinidad EM, et al. Chiari I malformation redefined: clinical and radiographic findings for 364 symptomatic patients. Neurosurgery 1999;44: 1005–17.

21. Garcia-Real I, Kass PH, Sturges BK, et al. Morphometric analysis of the cranial cavity and caudal cranial fossa in the dog: a computerized tomographic study. Vet Radiol Ultrasound 2004;45:38–45.

22. Schmidt MJ, Volk H, Klingler M, et al. Comparison of closure times for cranial base synchondroses in mesaticephalic, brachycephalic, and Cavalier King Charles Spaniel dogs. Vet Radiol Ultrasound 2013;54:497–503.

23. Couturier J, Rault D, Cauzinille L. Chiari-like malformation and syringomyelia in normal cavalier King Charles spaniels: a multiple diagnostic imaging approach. J Small Anim Pract 2008;49:438-43.
24. March PA, Berg JM, Smith M, et al. CSF flow abnormalities in caudal occipital malformation syndrome. J Vet Intern Med 2005;19:418-9.
25. Rusbridge C, Greitz D, Iskandar BJ. Syringomyelia: current concepts in pathogenesis, diagnosis, and treatment. J Vet Intern Med 2006;20:469-79.
26. Marmarou A, Shulman K, LaMorgese J. Compartmental analysis of compliance and outflow resistance of the cerebrospinal fluid system. J Neurosurg 1975;43: 523-34.
27. Rusbridge C, Jeffery ND. Pathophysiology and treatment of neuropathic pain associated with syringomyelia. Vet J 2008;175:164-72.
28. Driver CJ, Volk HA, Rusbridge C, et al. An update on the pathogenesis of syringomyelia secondary to Chiari-like malformations in dogs. Vet J 2013;198:551-9.
29. Cerda-Gonzalez S, Olby NJ, Broadstone R, et al. Characteristics of cerebrospinal fluid flow in Cavalier King Charles Spaniels analyzed using phase velocity cine magnetic resonance imaging. Vet Radiol Ultrasound 2009;50:467-76.
30. Fenn J, Schmidt MJ, Simpson H, et al. Venous sinus volume in the caudal cranial fossa in Cavalier King Charles spaniels with syringomyelia. Vet J 2013;197:896-7.
31. Schmidt MJ, Ondreka N, Sauerbrey M, et al. Volume reduction of the jugular foramina in Cavalier King Charles Spaniels with syringomyelia. BMC Vet Res 2012;8:158.
32. Milhorat TH, Capocelli AL Jr, Kotzen RM, et al. Intramedullary pressure in syringomyelia: clinical and pathophysiological correlates of syrinx distension. Neurosurgery 1997;41:1102-10.
33. Stoodley MA, Brown SA, Brown CJ, et al. Arterial pulsation-dependent perivascular cerebrospinal fluid flow into the central canal in the sheep spinal cord. J Neurosurg 1997;86:686-93.
34. Stoodley MA, Jones NR, Yang L, et al. Mechanisms underlying the formation and enlargement of noncommunicating syringomyelia: experimental studies. Neurosurg Focus 2000;8:E2.
35. Bilston LE, Stoodley MA, Fletcher DF. The influence of the relative timing of arterial and subarachnoid space pulse waves on spinal perivascular cerebrospinal fluid flow as a possible factor in syrinx development. J Neurosurg 2010;112:808-13.
36. Bagley R, Gavin P, Silver G, et al. Syringomyelia and hydromyelia in dogs and cats. Compend Contin Educ Pract Vet 2000;22:471-9.
37. Churcher RK, Child G. Chiari 1/syringomyelia complex in a King Charles Spaniel. Aust Vet J 2000;78:92-5.
38. Rusbridge C, MacSweeny JE, Davies JV, et al. Syringohydromyelia in Cavalier King Charles Spaniels. J Am Anim Hosp Assoc 2000;36:34-41.
39. Plessas IN, Rusbridge C, Driver CJ, et al. Long-term outcome of Cavalier King Charles spaniel dogs with clinical signs associated with Chiari-like malformation and syringomyelia. Vet Rec 2012;171:501.
40. Rusbridge C. Persistent scratching in Cavalier King Charles spaniels. Vet Rec 1997;141:179.
41. Hu HZ, Rusbridge C, Constantino-Casas F, et al. Histopathological investigation of syringomyelia in the Cavalier King Charles spaniel. J Comp Pathol 2012;146: 192-201.
42. Rusbridge C, Carruthers H, Dube M, et al. Syringomyelia in Cavalier King Charles spaniels: the relationship between syrinx dimensions and pain. J Small Anim Pract 2007;48:432-6.

43. Freeman AC, Platt SR, Kent M, et al. Chiari-like malformation and syringomyelia in American Brussels Griffon dogs. J Vet Intern Med 2014;28:1551–9.
44. Dewey CW, Berg JM, Barone G, et al. Foramen magnum decompression for treatment of caudal occipital malformation syndrome in dogs. J Am Vet Med Assoc 2005;227:1270–5, 1250–71.
45. Dewey CW, Marino DJ, Bailey KS, et al. Foramen magnum decompression with cranioplasty for treatment of caudal occipital malformation syndrome in dogs. Vet Surg 2007;36:406–15.
46. Dewey CW, Abramson CJ, Stefanacci JD, et al. Caudal occipital malformation syndrome in dogs. Compend Contin Educ Pract Vet 2004;26:886–95.
47. Child G, Higgins RJ, Cuddon PA. Acquired scoliosis associated with hydromyelia and syringomyelia in two dogs. J Am Vet Med Assoc 1986;189:909–12.
48. Tagaki S, Kadosawa T, Ohsaki T, et al. Hindbrain decompression in a dog with scoliosis associated with syringomyelia. J Am Vet Med Assoc 2005;226: 1359–63.
49. Graham KJ, Black AP, Brain PH. Resolution of life-threatening dysphagia caused by caudal occipital malformation syndrome following foramen magnum decompressive surgery. Aust Vet J 2012;90:297–300.
50. Dones J, De Jesus O, Colen CB, et al. Clinical outcomes in patients with Chiari I malformation: a review of 27 cases. Surg Neurol 2003;60:142–7 [discussion: 147–8].
51. Elta GH, Caldwell CA, Nostrant TT. Esophageal dysphagia as the sole symptom in type I Chiari malformation. Dig Dis Sci 1996;41:512–5.
52. Holschneider AM, Bliesener JA, Abel M. Brain stem dysfunction in Arnold-Chiari II syndrome [in German]. Z Kinderchir 1990;45:67–71.
53. Masson C, Colombani JM. Chiari type 1 malformation and magnetic resonance imaging [in French]. Presse Med 2005;34:1662–7.
54. Pollack IF, Pang D, Kocoshis S, et al. Neurogenic dysphagia resulting from Chiari malformations. Neurosurgery 1992;30:709–19.
55. Rusbridge C. Chiari-like malformation with syringomyelia in the Cavalier King Charles spaniel: long-term outcome after surgical management. Vet Surg 2007; 36:396–405.
56. Cole LK. Primary secretory otitis media in Cavalier King Charles spaniels. Vet Clin North Am Small Anim Pract 2012;42:1137–42.
57. Rusbridge C. Primary secretory otitis media in Cavalier King Charles spaniels. J Small Anim Pract 2004;45:222 [author reply: 222].
58. Stern-Berthholtz W, Sjostrom L, Wallin Hakanson N. Primary secretory otitis media in the Cavalier King Charles spaniel: a review of 61 cases. J Small Anim Pract 2003;44:253–6.
59. Loderstedt S, Benigni L, Chandler K, et al. Distribution of syringomyelia along the entire spinal cord in clinically affected Cavalier King Charles Spaniels. Vet J 2011; 190(3):359–63.
60. Iskandar BJ, Quigley M, Haughton VM. Foramen magnum cerebrospinal fluid flow characteristics in children with Chiari I malformation before and after craniocervical decompression. J Neurosurg 2004;101:169–78.
61. Kromhout K, van Bree H, Broeckx BJ, et al. Low-field MRI and multislice CT for the detection of cerebellar (foramen magnum) herniation in Cavalier King Charles Spaniels. J Vet Intern Med 2015;29:238–42.
62. Schmidt MJ, Wigger A, Jawinski S, et al. Ultrasonographic appearance of the craniocervical junction in normal brachycephalic dogs and dogs with caudal occipital (Chiari-like) malformation. Vet Radiol Ultrasound 2008;49: 472–6.

63. Bohn AA, Wills TB, West CL, et al. Cerebrospinal fluid analysis and magnetic resonance imaging in the diagnosis of neurologic disease in dogs: a retrospective study. Vet Clin Pathol 2006;35:315–20.
64. Itoh T, Nishimura R, Matsunaga S, et al. Syringomyelia and hydrocephalus in a dog. J Am Vet Med Assoc 1996;209:934–6.
65. Kirberger RM, Jacobson LS, Davies JV, et al. Hydromyelia in the dog. Vet Radiol Ultrasound 1997;38:30–8.
66. Hasegawa T, Taura Y, Kido H, et al. Surgical management of combined hydrocephalus, syringohydromyelia, and ventricular cyst in a dog. J Am Anim Hosp Assoc 2005;41:267–72.
67. Vermeersch K, Van Ham L, Caemaert J, et al. Suboccipital craniectomy, dorsal laminectomy of C1, durotomy and dural graft placement as a treatment for syringohydromyelia with cerebellar tonsil herniation in Cavalier King Charles spaniels. Vet Surg 2004;33:355–60.
68. Rusbridge C. Canine syringomyelia: a painful problem in man's best friend. Br J Neurosurg 2007;21:468–9.
69. Takahashi M, Kawaguchi M, Shimada K, et al. Systemic meloxicam reduces tactile allodynia development after L5 single spinal nerve injury in rats. Reg Anesth Pain Med 2005;30:351–5.
70. Bergh MS, Budsberg SC. The coxib NSAIDs: potential clinical and pharmacologic importance in veterinary medicine. J Vet Intern Med 2005;19:633–43.
71. Dembo G, Park SB, Kharasch ED. Central nervous system concentrations of cyclooxygenase-2 inhibitors in humans. Anesthesiology 2005;102:409–15.
72. Hamandi K, Sander JW. Pregabalin: a new antiepileptic drug for refractory epilepsy. Seizure 2006;15:73–8.
73. Moore RA, Straube S, Wiffen PJ, et al. Pregabalin for acute and chronic pain in adults. Cochrane Database Syst Rev 2009;(3):CD007076.
74. Salazar V, Dewey CW, Schwark W, et al. Pharmacokinetics of single-dose oral pregabalin administration in normal dogs. Vet Anaesth Analg 2009;36:574–80.
75. Gellman H. Reflex sympathetic dystrophy: alternatives modalities for pain management. Instr Course Lect 2000;49:549–57.
76. Giorgi M, Del Carlo S, Saccomanni G, et al. Biopharmaceutical profile of tramadol in the dog. Vet Res Commun 2009;33(Suppl 1):189–92.
77. Wood JN, Boorman JP, Okuse K, et al. Voltage-gated sodium channels and pain pathways. J Neurobiol 2004;61:55–71.
78. LaMont LA. Adjunctive analgesic therapy in veterinary medicine. Vet Clin North Am Small Anim Pract 2008;38:1187–203.
79. Gross AR, Dziengo S, Boers O, et al. Low level laser therapy (LLLT) for neck pain: a systematic review and meta-regression. Open Orthop J 2013;7:396–419.
80. Javaheri S, Corbett WS, Simbartl LA, et al. Different effects of omeprazole and Sch 28080 on canine cerebrospinal fluid production. Brain Res 1997;754:321–4.
81. Lindvall-Axelsson M, Nilsson C, Owman C, et al. Inhibition of cerebrospinal fluid formation by omeprazole. Exp Neurol 1992;115:394–9.
82. Carrion E, Hertzog JH, Medlock MD, et al. Use of acetazolamide to decrease cerebrospinal fluid production in chronically ventilated patients with ventriculopleural shunts. Arch Dis Child 2001;84:68–71.
83. Shinnar S, Gammon K, Bergman EW Jr, et al. Management of hydrocephalus in infancy: use of acetazolamide and furosemide to avoid cerebrospinal fluid shunts. J Pediatr 1985;107:31–7.

84. Vogh BP. The relation of choroid plexus carbonic anhydrase activity to cerebrospinal fluid formation: study of three inhibitors in cat with extrapolation to man. J Pharmacol Exp Ther 1980;213:321–31.

85. Artru AA, Powers KM. Furosemide decreases cerebrospinal fluid formation during desflurane anesthesia in rabbits. J Neurosurg Anesthesiol 1997;9:166–74.

86. Lorenzo AV, Hornig G, Zavala LM, et al. Furosemide lowers intracranial pressure by inhibiting CSF production. Z Kinderchir 1986;41(Suppl 1):10–2.

87. Pinegin LE, Dolzhenko DA, Natochin Iu V. Mechanism of the decrease in intracranial pressure as affected by furosemide [in Russian]. Biull Eksp Biol Med 1984; 98:682–5.

88. Vela AR, Carey ME, Thompson BM. Further data on the acute effect of intravenous steroids on canine CSF secretion and absorption. J Neurosurg 1979;50: 477–82.

89. Genitori L, Peretta P, Nurisso C, et al. Chiari type I anomalies in children and adolescents: minimally invasive management in a series of 53 cases. Childs Nerv Syst 2000;16:707–18.

90. Haroun RI, Guarnieri M, Meadow JJ, et al. Current opinions for the treatment of syringomyelia and chiari malformations: survey of the Pediatric Section of the American Association of Neurological Surgeons. Pediatr Neurosurg 2000;33: 311–7.

91. Krieger MD, McComb JG, Levy ML. Toward a simpler surgical management of Chiari I malformation in a pediatric population. Pediatr Neurosurg 1999;30:113–21.

92. Strayer A. Chiari I malformation: clinical presentation and management. J Neurosci Nurs 2001;33:90–6, 104.

93. Sakamoto H, Nishikawa M, Hakuba A, et al. Expansive suboccipital cranioplasty for the treatment of syringomyelia associated with Chiari malformation. Acta Neurochir (Wien) 1999;141:949–60 [discussion: 960–1].

94. Takayasu M, Takagi T, Hara M, et al. A simple technique for expansive suboccipital cranioplasty following foramen magnum decompression for the treatment of syringomyelia associated with Chiari I malformation. Neurosurg Rev 2004;27: 173–7.

95. Udani V, Holly LT, Chow D, et al. Posterior fossa reconstruction using titanium plate for the treatment of cerebellar ptosis after decompression for Chiari malformation. World Neurosurg 2014;81:836–41.

Atlantooccipital Overlap and Other Craniocervical Junction Abnormalities in Dogs

Catherine A. Loughin, DVM, Dominic J. Marino, DVM, CCRP*

KEYWORDS

- Atlantooccipital overlapping • Chiari-like malformation
- Craniocervical junction abnormalities • Syringomyelia • Dens angulation

KEY POINTS

- The term craniocervical junction abnormality (CJA), as used in human medicine, serves as an umbrella term for a variety of malformations that occur in the craniocervical region.
- MRI of craniocervical junction abnormalities with CT imaging are necessary to fully evaluate CJAs.
- Most dogs with atlantooccipital overlapping (AOO) respond temporarily to medical management. Like CLM/SM, we often consider AOO to be a surgical disorder.

Craniocervical junction abnormalities (CJA) are being recognized more frequently in veterinary patients. The term CJA is an umbrella term for a variety of malformations that occur in the craniocervical region. Chiari-like malformation (CLM) is commonly diagnosed in small-breed dogs, and is defined as an abnormal-shaped supraoccipital bone resulting in rostral compression of the caudal aspect of the cerebellum.[1–5] This is the most commonly diagnosed CJA, but other malformations include atlantooccipital overlapping (AOO),[6–8] atlantoaxial instability,[9–12] occipitoatlantoaxial malformation (OAAM),[13,14] atlantoaxial dural bands,[6–8,15] and dens abnormality.[6,16] Determining the structural cause of cerebellar compression is difficult on MRI because of poor bone visualization, but with the addition of computed tomography (CT) and three-dimensional reconstruction these structural abnormalities become easier to recognize.[8,17–19] Atlantoaxial instability and CLM are discussed elsewhere in this issue.

ATLANTOOCCIPITAL OVERLAPPING

AOO is a CJA recognized in small- and toy-breed dogs.[6,7,17] In this malformation, the atlas (C1) is cranially displaced into the foramen magnum, and overlap of the occipital

---

The authors have nothing to disclose.
Department of Surgery, Canine Chiari Institute, Long Island Veterinary Specialists, 163 South Service Road, Plainview, NY 11803, USA
* Corresponding author.
E-mail address: dmarino@livs.org

bone and the atlas occurs. This displacement tends to compress the caudal aspect of the cerebellum and to elevate and compress the caudal medulla (medullary kinking). AOO is likely a form of basilar invagination. Basilar invagination is a human craniocervical junction disorder where the atlas and/or the axis (C2) telescopes toward the foramen magnum.[20,21] One study found that nearly 30% of those diagnosed with CLM on MRI had AOO as the main CJA causing compression.[8] AOO can occur as a sole entity or in combination with CLM and/or atlantoaxial instability. Syringomyelia (SM) has frequently been associated with CLM and more recently with AOO; however, SM can occur as a sole malformation or as part of several craniocervical malformations in the same patient. Any CJA can disrupt the normal laminar flow of cerebrospinal fluid (CSF) in the subarachnoid space via compression secondarily creating SM. The typical age range for dogs with AOO at presentation seems to be broad; most dogs present by the time they are 4 years old (Loughin 2015, unpublished data). Toy-breeds, such as Yorkshire terriers and Chihuahuas, are diagnosed more frequently with AOO than CLM.[22]

Clinical signs in dogs with AOO typically include neck pain and varying degrees of ataxia of all four limbs.[6,7,17] As reported in the dogs with CLM, the most consistent clinical features also include cervical pain, pruritus of the head and neck, and cervical myelopathy making it impossible to distinguish CJAs based on clinical signs. Facial rubbing (pawing at the face and/or rubbing against objects) is also encountered in some dogs and is considered to be a form of pain and/or paresthesia. Spinal hyperpathia (typically cervical), scratching activity, and scoliosis are all generally believed to be related to interference of the syrinx cavity with ascending sensory pathways in the spinal cord. In a recent study it was found that Cavalier King Charles spaniel with AOO were more likely to have clinical signs compared with dogs with CLM (unpublished data).

Occasionally, dogs with AOO and cervical SM present with a specific variant of cervical myelopathy called central cord syndrome. In this scenario, the outwardly expanding syrinx in the cervicothoracic intumescence causes damage to the lower motor neurons of the thoracic limbs within the regional gray matter, leading to lower motor neuron paresis of the thoracic limbs, while sparing the more peripherally located white matter tracts (upper motor neurons to pelvic limbs). Damage to the regional white matter causes general proprioceptive/upper motor neuron paresis to the pelvic limbs. The result is thoracic limb paresis (lower motor neuron in nature) that is notably worse than pelvic limb paresis. In some dogs with this syndrome, the pelvic limbs may appear normal.[2,3,6,23]

Although the diagnosis of AOO can be made by MRI (**Fig 1**), which is also the preferred imaging modality for diagnosing CLM and SM, CT imaging (**Fig 2**) is extremely advantageous in assessing for the presence of CJAs. The precise nature of this and other CJAs is typically apparent on CT imaging. We routinely follow MRI of CJAs with CT imaging to fully evaluate the malformation or malformations in the region. A survey radiograph (**Fig 3**) may also reveal a CJA, such as AOO, but more advanced imaging gives more details of the soft tissue structures. On MRI, AOO is best visualized on a mid-sagittal view (preferably T2-weighted), which includes the caudal fossa and the cranial cervical spinal cord. Using the traditional MRI protocols for assessing CLM, dogs with AOO may have detectable malformation/malarticulation of the C1 and/or C2 vertebra and decreased distance between the cranial aspect of the dorsal spinous process of C2 and the occipital region. Because bony detail is difficult to distinguish on MRI, it is likely that AOO has been underdiagnosed in dogs, with most of these patients incorrectly ascribed a diagnosis of CLM.

We have found that some dogs with this malformation, similar to dogs with CLM/SM, respond to medical management (discussed elsewhere in this issue). Medical

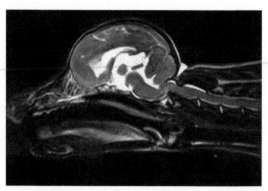

Fig. 1. T2-weighted sagittal MRI of a 2-year-old female spayed Yorkshire terrier with atlantooccipital overlap (*arrowhead*).

therapy for dogs with CJAs generally falls into three categories: (1) analgesic drugs (implies relief of dysesthesia/paresthesia also), (2) drugs that decrease CSF production in dogs with SM, and (3) corticosteroid therapy. In most cases of CJAs and SM, medical therapy diminishes the severity of clinical signs, but resolution is unlikely in most cases.[2,6,24,25] Both ventral and dorsal methods of stabilization of the atlantooccipital region have been described in people with basilar invagination with improvement in clinical signs.[26–28] AOO may also be managed in dogs with surgical stabilization.[17] The authors have successfully stabilized several AOO dogs using a ventral approach.

OCCIPITOATLANTOAXIAL MALFORMATIONS

OAAMs seldom occur in dogs, but they have been a well-recognized condition in the horse[13,14,29,30] and have been seen in humans, cows, cats, sheep, lions, camels, and a ferret.[14,31–35] These malformations include cervical vertebrae fusion, occipitoatlantal fusion, odontoid process and atlas hypoplasia, malformation of the axis, and atlantoaxial joint subluxation.[13,35] Variable degrees of spinal cord and brainstem compression occur secondary to malformed vertebrae or because of atlantoaxial instability.

Affected dogs are less than 2 years of age at the time clinical signs develop.[13,29] These malformations occur in small- and large-breed dogs, including Saint Bernard,

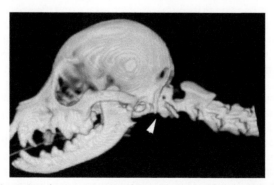

Fig. 2. A three-dimensional reconstruction from CT image of the same dog in **Fig. 1**. The *arrowhead* indicates the overlap.

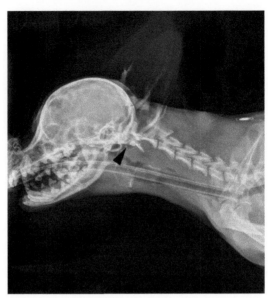

Fig. 3. A lateral head-cervical radiograph of the same dog in **Figs. 1** and **2**. The *arrowhead* indicates the overlap.

Cavalier King Charles spaniel, German shepherd, Jack Russell terrier, French bulldog, Newfoundland, and a Shiba Inu.[13,29] Clinical signs are typical of a cervical myelopathy: neck pain, proprioceptive deficits, ataxia, and tetraplegia.[13,29,35]

Occipitoatlantoaxial malformations are detectable on survey radiographs, but more details regarding the degree of spinal cord compression are assessed with myelography, CT, and MRI. The prognosis of OAAMs is considered guarded to poor, with many owners opting for euthanasia. Surgical stabilization of craniocervical junction has been described in three dogs with two of the dogs surviving the postoperative period and becoming ambulatory after the procedure.[29,36] Given the success of surgical stabilization with other CJAs, it may be proved to be beneficial in other cases of OAAM.

ATLANTOAXIAL DURAL BANDS

Dorsal fibrous bands have been described at the atlantooccipital and atlantoaxial junctions causing compression of the subarachnoid space and the spinal cord.[1,2,7,8,22] The degree of compression is variable, and has been noted in Cavalier King Charles spaniel and other small- and toy-breed dogs diagnosed with other CJAs, such as CLM, AOO, and atantoaxial instability.[6,8,15,22] In one study evaluating 274 small-breed dogs for CJAs, dorsal compression secondary to these bands was found in 38% of the dogs.[8] This band of tissue arises from the dura or interarcuate ligament, and is composed of areas of lymphoplasmacytic inflammation and fibrosis with mineralization, osseous metaplasia, or both.[2,22,37] It is believed that chronic instability at C1/2 junction leads to the formation of these bands.

Diagnosis of dural bands is best noted on T2-weighted sagittal MRI (**Fig 4**). Dilation of the subarachnoid space cranial and caudal to the lesion may also be seen on these images.[1,8,15,38] In one study it was noted that the atlantoaxial dural band was more prominent in extended views of the cervical region than in flexed positions.[15] Presence of these bands in humans with Chiari malformation (CM) has been found to play an

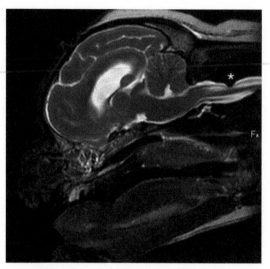

Fig. 4. T2-weighted sagittal MRI of an 8-year-old male neutered Boston terrier with atlantoaxial dorsal compression from fibrous bands (*asterisk*).

important role in the development of clinical signs and SM.[37,39] In dogs with CJAs, neuropathic pain and development of SM have been associated with increasing severity of dorsal compression secondary to dorsal bands. Clinical signs of cervical myelopathy have also been noted.[7,8,15,22,38]

Treatment involves resection of the tissue at the time of primary decompression for a corresponding CJA. Removal of this band reestablishes CSF flow to the subarachnoid space and can lead to improvement in clinical signs.[7,22] Recognition of these dural bands during diagnosis and including their removal in the surgical plan can improve the overall prognosis.

DENS ABNORMALITIES

Dens abnormalities are likely secondary to abnormal development. Ischemic necrosis of the dens and absence of a dens ossification center are proposed mechanisms for

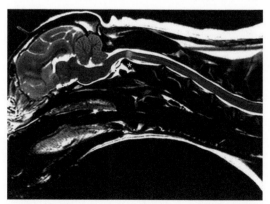

Fig. 5. T2-weighted sagittal MRI of a 2-year-old female spayed Cavalier King Charles spaniel with dorsal angulation of the dens (*asterisk*).

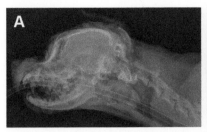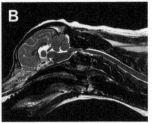

Fig. 6. Postoperative lateral radiograph (*A*) and T2-weighted sagittal MRI (*B*) of the same dog in **Fig. 6**. This dog had a foramen magnum decompression with cranioplasty and a ventral stabilization of C1-2.

dens agenesis/hypoplasia. Congenital nonunion and dorsal angulation of the dens are also documented abnormalties.[7,16,40–43] Like other CJAs, dens abnormalities occur most commonly in small- and toy-breed dogs, but there have been a few reports in large-breed dogs.[44–46]

Dorsal angulation of the dens decreases the vertebral canal diameter and compresses the spinal cord causing kinking of the brainstem. This alters CSF dynamics and blood flow, and causes signs of compressive myelopathy. Clinical signs may be static or progressive, and include neck pain, ataxia, tetraparesis, and proprioceptive deficits. A hypermetric gait may be seen secondary to compression of the spinocerebellar tract. Angulation of the dens is seen on lateral cervical radiographs, CT, and MRI (**Fig 5**) with secondary spinal cord compression noted on CT and MRI. Three-dimensional reconstruction of CT images can clarify the abnormality if radiographs are unclear. Dorsal angulation of the dens has been documented in human CM, more specifically in female patients, and recently was documented in 66% to 68% of small-breed dogs evaluated for CLM.[1,8]

Treatment involves decompression of the spinal cord and brainstem compression. Odontoidectomy has been reported,[43,47,48] and fusion of the atlantoaxial joint.[11] Recommendations for humans with CM and dens angulation include decompression of the brainstem by ventral cervical spinal fusion to lessen cervical spinal cord injury followed by foramen magnum decompression.[49] A clinical study is in progress to assess the results of ventral decompression and stabilization with foramen magnum decompression with cranioplasty in dogs with CLM, AOO, and dorsal angulation of the dens (**Fig 6**).

SUMMARY

CJAs are commonly diagnosed in small- and toy-breed dogs with signs of pain and cervical myelopathy. Even though CLM may be the most commonly diagnosed CJA, other CJAs can occur concomitantly with CLM in dogs predisposed to CJAs and should be considered and evaluated for before treatment plans are devised. MRI is the best modality for diagnosis, but CT and radiographs can also play a role. Medical management is beneficial for some dogs, but surgery benefits most dogs diagnosed.

REFERENCES

1. Cerda-Gonzalez S, Olby NJ, McCullough S, et al. Morphology of the caudal fossa in Cavalier King Charles spaniels. Vet Radiol Ultrasound 2009;50:37–46.

2. Dewey CW, Berg JM, Barone G, et al. Foramen magnum decompression for treatment of caudal occipital malformation syndrome in dogs. J Am Vet Med Assoc 2005;227:1270–5, 1250–71.
3. Dewey CW, Marino DJ, Bailey KS, et al. Foramen magnum decompression with cranioplasty for treatment of caudal occipital malformation syndrome in dogs. Vet Surg 2007;36:406–15.
4. Dewey CW, Berg JM, Stefanacci JD, et al. Caudal occipital malformation syndrome in dogs. Compend Contin Educ Pract Vet 2004;26:886–95.
5. Rusbridge C. Chiari-like malformation with syringomyelia in the Cavalier King Charles spaniel: long-term outcome after surgical management. Vet Surg 2007; 36:396–405.
6. Cerda-Gonzalez S, Dewey CW. Congenital diseases of the craniocervical junction in the dog. Vet Clin North Am Small Anim Pract 2010;40:121–41.
7. Cerda-Gonzalez S, Dewey CW, Scrivani PV, et al. Imaging features of atlanto-occipital overlapping in dogs. Vet Radiol Ultrasound 2009;50:264–8.
8. Marino DJ, Loughin CA, Dewey CW, et al. Morphometric features of the craniocervical junction region in dogs with suspected Chiari-like malformation determined by combined use of magnetic resonance imaging and computed tomography. Am J Vet Res 2012;73:105–11.
9. LeCouteur RA, McKeown D, Johnson J, et al. Stabilization of atlantoaxial subluxation in the dog, using the nuchal ligament. J Am Vet Med Assoc 1980;177:1011–7.
10. McCarthy RJ, Lewis DD, Hosgood G. Atlantoaxial subluxation in dogs. Compendium 1995;17:215–27.
11. Platt SR, Chambers JN, Cross A. A modified ventral fixation for surgical management of atlantoaxial subluxation in 19 dogs. Vet Surg 2004;33:349–54.
12. Watson AG, de Lahunta A. Atlantoaxial subluxation and absence of transverse ligament of the atlas in a dog. J Am Vet Med Assoc 1989;195:235–7.
13. Petite A, McConnell F, De Stefani A, et al. Congenital occipito-atlanto-axial malformation in five dogs. Vet Radiol Ultrasound 2009;50:118.
14. Watson AG, de Lahunta A, Evans HE. Morphology and embryological interpretation of a congenital occipito-atlanto-axial malformation in a dog. Teratology 1988; 38:451–9.
15. Cerda-Gonzalez S, Olby NJ, Griffith EH. Dorsal compressive atlantoaxial bands and the craniocervical junction syndrome: association with clinical signs and syringomyelia in mature cavalier King Charles spaniels. J Vet Intern Med 2015;29: 887–92.
16. Parker AJ, Park RD, Cusick PK. Abnormal odontoid process angulation in a dog. Vet Rec 1973;93:559–61.
17. Dewey CW, Cerda-Gonzalez S, Scrivani PV, et al. Surgical stabilization of a craniocervical junction abnormality with atlanto-occipital overlapping in a dog. Compend Contin Educ Vet 2009;31(10):E1–6.
18. Rylander H, Robles JC. Diagnosis and treatment of a chronic atlanto-occipital subluxation in a dog. J Am Anim Hosp Assoc 2007;43:173–8.
19. Steffen F, Flueckiger M, Montavon PM. Traumatic atlanto-occipital luxation in a dog: associated hypoglossal nerve deficits and use of 3-dimensional computed tomography. Vet Surg 2003;32:411–5.
20. Goel A, Bhatjiwale M, Desai K. Basilar invagination: a study based on 190 surgically treated patients. J Neurosurg 1998;88:962–8.
21. Pearce JM. Platybasia and basilar invagination. Eur Neurol 2007;58:62–4.
22. Dewey CW, Marino DJ, Loughin CA. Craniocervical junction abnormalities in dogs. N Z Vet J 2013;61:202–11.

23. Rusbridge C, Carruthers H, Dube M, et al. Syringomyelia in Cavalier King Charles spaniels: the relationship between syrinx dimensions and pain. J Small Anim Pract 2007;48:432–6.
24. Rusbridge C, Dewey C. Treatment of canine Chiari-like malformation and syringomyelia. In: Bonagura J, Twedt D, editors. Kirk's current veterinary therapy. Philadelphia: Saunders; 2009. p. 1102.
25. Dewey CW, Berg JM, Barone G, et al. Treatment of caudal occipital malformation syndrome in dogs by foramen decompression. J Vet Intern Med 2005;19:418.
26. Goel A. Treatment of basilar invagination by atlantoaxial joint distraction and direct lateral mass fixation. J Neurosurg Spine 2004;1:281–6.
27. Goel A, Sharma P. Craniovertebral junction realignment for the treatment of basilar invagination with syringomyelia: preliminary report of 12 cases. Neurol Med Chir (Tokyo) 2005;45:512–7 [discussion: 518].
28. Schultz KD Jr, Petronio J, Haid RW, et al. Pediatric occipitocervical arthrodesis. A review of current options and early evaluation of rigid internal fixation techniques. Pediatr Neurosurg 2000;33:169–81.
29. Galban EM, Gilley RS, Long SN. Surgical stabilization of an occipitoatlantoaxial malformation in an adult dog. Vet Surg 2010;39:1001–4.
30. Rosenstein DS, Schott HC 2nd, Stickle RL. Imaging diagnosis–occipitoatlantoaxial malformation in a miniature horse foal. Vet Radiol Ultrasound 2000;41:218–9.
31. Bell S, Detweiler D, Benak J, et al. What is your diagnosis? Occipitoatlantoaxial malformation. J Am Vet Med Assoc 2007;231:1033–4.
32. De Castro N, Barreiro JD, Espino L. What is your diagnosis? Congenital occipitoatlantoaxial malformation. J Am Vet Med Assoc 2014;245:631–3.
33. Watson AC, Coke RL, Rochat MC, et al. Congenital occipitoatlantoaxial malformation in a cat. Compend Contin Educ Pract Vet 1985;7:245–52.
34. Galloway DS, Coke RL, Rochat MC, et al. Spinal compression due to atlantal vertebral malformation in two African lions (Panthera leo). J Zoo Wildl Med 2002;33:249–55.
35. Watson AG, Wilson JH, Cooley AJ, et al. Occipito-atlanto-axial malformation with atlanto-axial subluxation in an ataxic calf. J Am Vet Med Assoc 1985;187:740–2.
36. Read R, Brett S, Cahill J. Surgical treatment of occipito-atlanto-axial malformation in the dog. Aust Vet Pract 1987;4:184–9.
37. Nakamura N, Iwasaki Y, Hida K, et al. Dural band pathology in syringomyelia with Chiari type I malformation. Neuropathology 2000;20:38–43.
38. Tagaki S, Kadosawa T, Ohsaki T, et al. Hindbrain decompression in a dog with scoliosis associated with syringomyelia. J Am Vet Med Assoc 2005;226:1359–63.
39. Hida K, Iwasaki Y, Koyanagi I, et al. Surgical indication and results of foramen magnum decompression versus syringosubarachnoid shunting for syringomyelia associated with Chiari I malformation. Neurosurgery 1995;37:673–8 [discussion: 678–9].
40. Bailey CS, Morgan JP. Congenital spinal malformations. Vet Clin North Am Small Anim Pract 1992;22:985–1015.
41. Bynevelt M, Rusbridge C, Britton J. Dorsal dens angulation and a Chiari type malformation in a Cavalier King Charles spaniel. Vet Radiol Ultrasound 2000;41:521–4.
42. Ladds P, Guffy M, Blauch B, et al. Congenital odontoid process separation in two dogs. J Small Anim Pract 1971;12:463–71.
43. Swaim S, Greene C. Odontoidectomy in a dog. J Am Anim Hosp Assoc 1975;11: 663.
44. Patton KM, Almes KM, de Lahunta A. Absence of the dens in a 9.5-year-old Rottweiler with non-progressive clinical signs. Can Vet J 2010;51:1007–10.

45. Stigen O, Aleksandersen M, Sorby R, et al. Acute non-ambulatory tetraparesis with absence of the dens in two large breed dogs: case reports with a radiographic study of relatives. Acta Vet Scand 2013;55:31.
46. Wheeler SJ. Atlantoaxial subluxation with absence of dens in a Rottweiler. J Small Anim Pract 1992;33:90–3.
47. Sorjonen DC, Shires PK. Atlantoaxial instability: a ventral surgical technique for decompression, fixation, and fusion. Vet Surg 1981;10:22–9.
48. Thomas WB, Sorjonen DC, Simpson ST. Surgical management of atlantoaxial subluxation in 23 dogs. Vet Surg 1991;20:409–12.
49. Kubota M, Yamauchi T, Saeki N. Surgical results of foramen magnum decompression for Chiari type 1 malformation associated with syringomyelia: a retrospective study on neuroradiological characters influencing shrinkage of syringes. Spinal Surg 2004;18:81–6.

Intracranial Intra-arachnoid Diverticula and Cyst-like Abnormalities of the Brain

Simon Platt, BVM&S, MRCVS[a],*, Jill Hicks, DVM[b],
Lara Matiasek, DrMedVet, MRCVS[c]

KEYWORDS

- Intracranial • Arachnoid • Cysts • Dogs • MRI

KEY POINTS

- Intracranial cysts are classically lesions with an epithelial lining filled with fluid.
- If a cyst has an incomplete epithelial lining it is called a diverticula.
- The most common primary congenital intracranial cysts are intra-arachnoid, dermoid, and epidermoid.
- Intracranial cysts cause clinical signs directly by compressing local brain tissue.
- Diagnosis is often possible with advanced imaging techniques, such as MRI.

INTRODUCTION

Intracranial cysts are classically lesions with an epithelial lining filled with fluid that can directly cause clinical signs from compression of the brain or indirectly by producing obstructive hydrocephalus.[1,2] Intracranial cysts may enlarge by secreting cerebrospinal fluid (CSF) into the cyst, by way of an osmotic gradient depending on the cyst contents, or by exfoliation of cyst lining or materials into the lumen.[1,2] Cystic lesions of the brain are easily recognized on MRI and computed tomography (CT) scanning by way of their morphologic features, which include a rounded shape, well-defined borders, size, and cyst wall thickness. Further characterization is possible based on their radiographic attenuation properties on CT scans or by their signal intensity on MRI.[2,3]

The authors have nothing to disclose.
[a] Neurology and Neurosurgery Service, Department of Small Animal Medicine and Surgery, College of Veterinary Medicine, University of Georgia, 2200 College Station Road, Athens, GA 30602, USA; [b] Department of Small Animal Medicine and Surgery, College of Veterinary Medicine, University of Georgia, 2200 College Station Road, Athens, GA 30602, USA; [c] Neurology Referral Service, Tierklinik Haar, Keferloher Strasse 25, 85540 Haar, Germany
* Corresponding author.
E-mail address: srplatt@uga.edu

Vet Clin Small Anim 46 (2016) 253–263
http://dx.doi.org/10.1016/j.cvsm.2015.10.004
0195-5616/16/$ – see front matter © 2016 Elsevier Inc. All rights reserved.
vetsmall.theclinics.com

INTRACRANIAL INTRA-ARACHNOID DIVERTICULA

Intracranial intra-arachnoid cyst-like lesions represent accumulations of CSF that occur because of splitting or duplication of the arachnoid membrane.[4,5] Because in some cases there is no evidence of a complete encapsulating membrane in which case the fluid is surrounded by normal tissue, the lesions are more appropriately termed diverticula.[6] These diverticulae constitute 1% of all nontraumatic, space-occupying intracranial lesions in human adults[7] and occur in 2.6% of children,[8] with supratentorial and infratentorial locations.[9] In dogs, more than 60 cases of intracranial intra-arachnoid diverticula (IADs) have been reported, all located within the caudal fossa; most seem to occur in a region comparable with the quadrigeminal cistern in humans, and therefore have often been called quadrigeminal cysts.[5,10–21] An extensive review of canine MRI brain scans documented a low prevalence of the condition, with 0.7% of dogs being screened for brain disease affected.[19]

Pathophysiology

It has been postulated that during embryonic development the perimedullary mesh experiences a splitting in the arachnoid layer because of aberrant CSF flow; this mesh surrounds the developing neural tube and is normally divided by CSF flow into the pia and arachnoid layers.[18] Evaluation of the lining of these cysts has determined there to be multiple structural variants, which may explain their differential clinical behavior.[22] Secondary intracranial IADs can also occur and represent acquired accumulations of CSF that result from loculation of the subarachnoid space resulting from head injury, intracranial infection/inflammation, neoplasia, or hemorrhage, and are surrounded by arachnoid scarring rather than normal arachnoid tissue.[14,18,23]

The mechanism by which a cyst expands is controversial. There is some evidence that the lining of the cyst wall may have secretory abilities; however, many cysts do not enlarge and can even resolve, which implies that this cannot be universal in all patients.[24] Additionally, a one-way or "ball-valve" effect has been hypothesized and there has been evidence of one-way flow suggested by cine MRI with confirmation of a slit-valve structure confirmed via endoscopy.[25,26]

Three heterogeneous phenotypes of IAD (quadrigeminal) have been described in dogs: they can appear associated with either the third or fourth ventricle, or may have a loculated appearance and be associated with both third and fourth ventricles.[19] The heterogeneous appearance and lack of a true "cyst" wall has led some to refer to them as supracollicular fluid accumulations instead of IADs.[19] The association found between ventricles in some of these cysts must not be confused with the term communicating and noncommunicating IADs, because this refers to their communication with the subarachnoid space,[7,18,26] which cannot be determined with conventional imaging.

Clinical Signs

Small breed brachycephalic male dogs seem to be predisposed to IADs with the most common breed reported being the Shih Tzu.[10,11,14,16–20] Subarachnoid diverticula have been reported within the fourth ventricle in five nonbrachycephalic large breed dogs, indicating that the brachycephalic predisposition may only occur for IADs in dogs. Age at presentation varies widely, and is likely related to whether the IAD is incidental or contributes to clinical signs along with another intracranial disease. The onset of clinical signs in elderly patients has been reported with intracystic hemorrhage occurring after trauma.[9,14] Variable clinical significance of IADs is reported for humans and dogs. They might be an incidental imaging or postmortem finding[18,19,23,27–29] or give rise to severe neurologic dysfunction.[5,11,15,16,18–21,23,27,29,30] In more than half of dogs retrospectively evaluated for intracranial disease, an IAD was considered an incidental finding.[19] Clinical signs that were attributable to the cysts in this study included focal or generalized seizures and cerebellar/vestibulocerebellar signs; however paresis, a reduced level of consciousness, facial nerve paresis, and neck pain have also been reported.[5,10,11,14–21,30] Overall, clinical signs reflect the location of the cyst and most likely occur as a result of compression of the neural tissue. Based on an MRI study, occipital lobe compression greater than 14% is likely to cause clinical signs, whereas the degree of cerebellar compression is not significantly associated with the occurrence of clinical signs.[19] Seizures and headaches are the most common clinical signs in humans, probably because of the more common[23] supratentorial location of the diverticulae[23]; hydrocephalus secondary to obstruction of the mesencephalic aqueduct by the lesion is an important pathologic mechanism that can lead to clinical signs, such as seizures, mental retardation, and headaches.[8,23,27–29,31] This is not commonly documented in dogs and has only been reported rarely.[18,19] Some investigators believe that the breed predisposition for ventriculomegaly, where observed, is the same as the predisposition for IADs, indicating that these two developmental disorders may have a common cause given that there is inadequate evidence that the diverticula are the cause of hydrocephalus in dogs affected with both.[19]

Diagnosis

CT, MRI, and ultrasonography have all been described as imaging modalities used to assist in the diagnosis of IADs in veterinary medicine[5,14–17,19–21,30] (Fig. 1). Typical imaging characteristics include (1) extra-axial, midline, frequently supracollicular location; (2) fluid similar in appearance to that of CSF; and (3) lack of contrast enhancement of the tissue immediately surrounding the fluid on MRI or CT.[18] A hypointense fluid-filled structure on T1-weighted images, which is hyperintense on T2-weighted images and fully suppresses with fluid-attenuated inversion recovery (FLAIR) imaging, is typically seen on MRI.[5,16,30] Hemorrhage into the lumen of these cysts has been documented to have a signal intensity that is mixed or hyperintense to CSF in T1-weighted images and isointense to hypointense to CSF on T2-weighted images with lack of suppression on FLAIR.[9,14] The appearance of intracystic hemorrhage varies with its age, amount, hemoglobin oxygen state, and the strength of the magnetic field, but gradient echo images may aid in diagnosis.[9,14] If intraluminal hemorrhage has occurred, the diverticula may be difficult to visualize with CT images, because of the similar attenuation characteristics to the brain parenchyma; however, hemorrhage

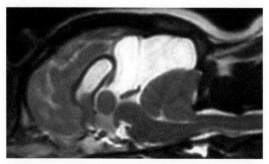

Fig. 1. A mid-line sagittal T2-weighted MRI of the brain of a 1-year-old German shepherd dog. Note the hyperintense cyst-like structure in the quadrigeminal cistern, which is deviating the cerebellum caudally.

can settle to dependent areas, which may result in a blood-CSF interface.[14] Transcranial ultrasonography of these lesions represents a noninvasive manner in which to monitor cysts and/or associated ventriculomegaly; this has been reported in three dogs, with the cyst contents being anechoic and the images being obtained via the temporal window or the foramen magnum where a persistent fontanelle does not exist. Characterization with CT cisternograms or ventriculograms[7] or phase-contrast cine MRI has been evaluated as extremely reliable for presurgical diagnosis of communicating IADs in humans.[7,26]

Treatment

The main treatment options for IADs considered to be either the primary or contributory cause of clinical signs in dogs are cyst wall fenestration or placement of a cyst-peritoneal shunt.[14,15,17,18,20,21] The role of medical therapy is not yet clear for clinically affected animals.[5,18] Craniotomy with cyst resection and endoscopically assisted fenestration has been very successful in humans.[8,23,27,29,32] However, considering that IADs are often an incidental imaging finding in dogs and humans,[19,28] other causes of neurologic signs should be ruled out before considering surgical intervention.[18]

EPIDERMOID CYSTS

Intracranial epidermoid cysts are rare lesions also known as cholesteatomas. In humans, these cysts constitute approximately 1% of intracranial masses.[33] There are sporadic case reports of affected dogs that represent postmortem findings and only occasionally include attempted therapy.[34–41] Most of the intracranial canine epidermoid cysts reported have been located in the cerebellopontine/medullary angle, and can extend into the fourth ventricle[34,35,37–42] (**Fig. 2**). This neuroanatomic location is also the most common site of human intracranial epidermoid cysts and is thought to be related to the sequence of neural tube closure.[33] An extradural location has been reported in about 10% of human epidermoid cysts, but this has not yet been reported in dogs.[2]

Pathophysiology

These cystic lesions are congenital and of ectodermal origin, believed to be formed by aberrant inclusion of nonneural ectoderm with the neural tube.[34,36] Epidermoid cysts are lined by stratified squamous epithelium and contain keratinocytes, keratinaceous debris, and cholesterol.[34] The stratified squamous epithelium lining of epidermal cysts is believed to undergo progressive exfoliation leading to an accumulation of keratinized material, cholesterol clefts, and some inflammatory cells in the lumen and subsequent expansion of the cyst.[2,42,43] The lining of the epidermoid cyst helps differentiate these structures from dermoid cysts, which have a more complex arrangement of dermis that may include hair follicles, sebaceous glands, and sweat glands.[2,37,42]

Clinical Signs

Neurologic signs were not reported in several dogs with central nervous system epidermoid cysts; the cyst was an incidental finding on postmortem examination[38,40,42]; because the cysts show slow, linear growth, neurologic signs often present in middle age in humans and dogs.[33–36,43,44] Because of the common location of epidermoid cysts in the cerebellopontine/medullary angle, vestibular signs are frequently reported in humans and dogs[33–36,41–45] with up to 93% of human patients presenting with CN VIII dysfunction in one study.[46] Besides signs attributable to the space-occupying nature of the cysts, secondary complications have also been reported in humans including

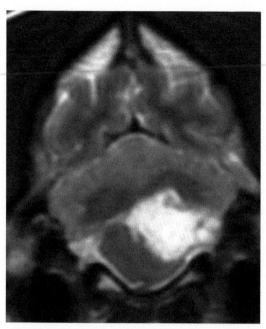

Fig. 2. A transverse T2-weighted MRI of the brain of an 18-month-old English setter at the level of the caudal fossa. There is an irregularly defined hyperintense lesion with mass effect in the cerebellomedullary pontine angle. This was surgically removed and histopathology confirmed an epidermoid cyst.

chemical meningitis, malignant transformation into squamous cell carcinoma, and foreign body giant cell reactions.[33,43,45,47] Chemical meningitis can be caused by the release of keratin/cholesterol breakdown products into the CSF as a result of spontaneous cyst rupture or following biopsy or subtotal resection.[34,43,44,47] Protein and total cell count elevations in the CSF have been recorded in some dogs with epidermoid cysts, which may represent chemical meningitis in those cases; however, chemical meningitis specifically associated with an epidermoid cyst has only been reported in one dog.[36,48]

Diagnosis

The MRI appearance of epidermoid cysts tends to be similar to CSF on T2- and T1-weighted imaging, although there may be heterogeneity in the appearance secondary to cellular debris within the cyst[33,35,36,49,50] (see **Fig. 2**). The cysts can often be hyperintense on T2- and T1-weighted imaging.[2] FLAIR suppression is typically incomplete; there may be a thin rim of cyst wall contrast enhancement, and on diffusion-weighted imaging there is often restricted diffusion compared with CSF because of the cellular debris within the cyst fluid; these features help to differentiate epidermoid cysts from intra-arachnoid diverticulae.[2,33,50] Hydrocephalus has not been reported frequently in conjunction with epidermoid cysts, but is possible if cyst location causes obstruction as described in two published reports of dogs with cysts in the fourth ventricle.[34,36] The cysts often have a lobulated appearance, with a smooth "mother-of-pearl" sheen grossly.[2] On CT, these cysts in humans are often well-demarcated, hypoattenuating lesions that do not enhance with contrast media and may have calcification present.[2] Only one CT case report in a dog exists and describes the epidermoid cyst as a homogenous, hypoattenuating mass with slight peripheral ring enhancement.[36]

Treatment

The goal for treatment in humans is to totally resect these cysts when possible because of the high recurrence rate of subtotally resected epidermoid cysts.[44,51] Postoperative aseptic (chemical) meningitis has been reported in between 2% and 50% of human patients.[43] Recurrence rate varies significantly with total versus subtotal resection at 9% versus 93% on long-term follow-up.[51] One of the authors has successfully removed an epidermoid cyst from the cerebellomedullary pontine angle of a dog, with good long-term resolution of clinical signs. Adjunctive therapy, such as radiation or chemotherapy, is only considered potentially beneficial in cases with malignant transformation, which has not been reported in dogs.[45]

DERMOID CYSTS

Intracranial dermoid cysts are more infrequent than epidermoid cysts in human and veterinary medicine, with only two cases reported in dogs to the authors' knowledge.[52,53] These cysts represent an estimated maximum of 0.6% of intracranial masses in humans.[54]

Pathophysiology

The cyst walls of these benign lesions contain epidermoid tissue and adnexa, which can include hair follicles, sebaceous, apocrine, and sweat glands.[54] They are formed in a similar manner to epidermoid cysts and are most commonly located in the caudal fossa on the midline in humans and in dogs.[52–56]

Diagnosis

Intracranial dermoid cysts have a heterogeneous MRI appearance; there is predominantly a hyperintense signal on T1- and T2-weighting because of the presence of variable amounts of fat.[2] Any visible hypointensity is attributed to the presence of calcification, glandular tissue, sweat, or hair, the latter described as curvilinear inclusions within the mass.[54,57] Contrast enhancement has not been reported, and the masses do not seem to be associated with surrounding edema.[2] A medullary dermoid cyst in a dog has been described as a roughly spherical mass with a predominantly hyperintense signal on T1- and T2-weighted imaging; the lesion did not contrast enhance[52] (**Fig. 3**). Intracranial dermoid cysts can be associated with an obstructive hydrocephalus in dogs and humans because of their typical location.[2,52,54] The CT appearance of these cysts in humans is hypoattenuating, typical of fat, with a more or less heterogeneous appearance depending on the degree of adnexal content.[2,58] Dermoid cyst rupture is diagnosed by the presence of "droplets" with the imaging characteristics of fat within the subarachnoid space, ventricles, or sulci,[2,52,54,58] resulting in aseptic meningitis, as with epidermoid cysts[52,58]; a susceptibility artifact similar to that of hemorrhage can appear on susceptibility-weighted imaging in patients with ruptured cysts.[52,54,58,59]

Treatment

Treatment of intracranial dermoid cysts is as for epidermoids, with likelihood of recurrence if the mass cannot be completely resected.[55] Ventriculoperitoneal shunting is performed in human and canine patients with an associated hydrocephalus.[52,54,58]

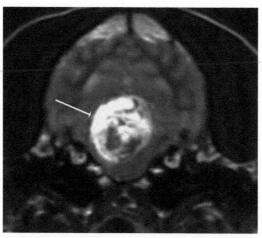

Fig. 3. A transverse T2-weighted MRI of the brain of a 5-year, 8-month old Springer spaniel at the level of the caudal fossa. A dermoid cyst is shown here (*arrow*) as a heterogeneous hyperintense lesion within the parenchyma of the cerebellum.

CHOROID PLEXUS CYSTS

Choroid plexus cysts (CPCs) are rare in humans and have only been reported twice in dogs to the authors' knowledge.[2,60,61] These cysts are frequently bilateral and found in the atria of the lateral ventricles, although occasionally reported in the third ventricle.[2,62,63]

Pathophysiology

Formation of CPCs is believed to occur by "infolding" of the choroid epithelial lining into fluid-filled structures; another theory proposed describes lipid accumulation within the choroid plexus leading to cyst formation.[2,60] A clear CSF-like substance is produced within these cysts, which may cause the cysts to expand to a clinically important size, although typically they remain small[2,63,64]; this is caused by the absorptive and secretory properties of the choroid plexus.

Clinical Signs

A clinical syndrome is rarely associated with CPCs unless obstructive hydrocephalus occurs, typically because of obstruction of the interventricular foramen; in humans, CPCs are most frequently found incidentally in adults or during ultrasound screening in neonates,[2,60,62,64] although sporadic reports exist of CPCs forming secondary to trauma or after surgical shunting.[65,66]

Diagnosis

CT and MRI studies of CPCs have been reported in humans and dogs.[2,60,61] CT findings in humans describe the cysts as isoattenuating to hyperattenuating in nonenhanced images, whereas the report in a dog described a hypoattenuating lesion with mild peripheral enhancement.[2,61] In humans MRI characteristics of CPCs are similar to those of CSF, although the lesions may be hyperintense to CSF on T2- and T1-weighted images. FLAIR suppression is often incomplete because of elevated protein concentration within the cysts; either rim or homogenous contrast enhancement is often seen.[2] The only reported MRI study of a CPC in a dog described T2-weighted hyperintensity;

T1-weighted hypointensity; and strong, homogenous contrast enhancement.[60] Contrast enhancement maybe related to vascularity of the cysts, but the cause of homogenous enhancement is not described.

SUMMARY

Primary intracranial cystic or cyst-like lesions include intra-arachnoid diverticula, epidermoid, dermoid, and CPCs. Differentiation of these cystic lesions can usually be accomplished by imaging studies alone; however, some cysts are similar in appearance and require histopathology for definitive diagnosis. Clinical signs often reflect the location of the cysts within the intracranial cavity rather than the type of cyst. If clinical signs are significant and progressive, surgical removal is warranted and may be successful, although cystic contents could be harmful if allowed to contact surrounding brain parenchyma or meninges.

REFERENCES

1. Osborn A. Miscellaneous tumors, cysts, and metastases. Diagnostic neuroradiology. St Louis (MO): Mosby; 1994. p. 631–49.
2. Osborn AG, Preece MT. Intracranial cysts: radiologic-pathologic correlation and imaging approach 1. Radiology 2006;239:650–64.
3. MacKillop E. Magnetic resonance imaging of intracranial malformations in dogs and cats. Vet Radiol Ultrasound 2011;52:S42–51.
4. Vernau KM, Kortz GD, Koblik PD, et al. Magnetic resonance imaging and computed tomography characteristics of intracranial intra-arachnoid cysts in 6 dogs. Vet Radiol Ultrasound 1997;38:171–6.
5. Min-Hee K, Suk-Won L, Hyung-Joong K, et al. Serial magnetic resonance imaging and long-term medical management of intracranial arachnoid cyst in a dog. Pak Vet J 2014;34:417–9.
6. Bazelle J, Caine A, Palus V, et al. MRI characteristics of fourth ventricle arachnoid diverticula in five dogs. Vet Radiol Ultrasound 2015;56:196–203.
7. Wang X, Chen JX, You C, et al. CT cisternography in intracranial symptomatic arachnoid cysts: classification and treatment. J Neurol Sci 2012;318:125–30.
8. Ali ZS, Lang S-S, Bakar D, et al. Pediatric intracranial arachnoid cysts: comparative effectiveness of surgical treatment options. Childs Nerv Syst 2014;30:461–9.
9. Arora R, Puligopu AK, Uppin MS, et al. Suprasellar arachnoid cyst with spontaneous intracystic hemorrhage: a rare complication. Role of MR and illustration of a case. Pol J Radiol 2014;79:422–5.
10. Nagae H, Oomura T, Kato Y. A disorder resembling arachnoid cyst in a dog. J Jpn Vet Neurol 1995;2:9–14.
11. Orima H, Fujita M, Hara Y. A case of the dog with arachnoid cyst. Jpn J Vet Imag 1998;10:49–51.
12. Koie H, Kitagawa M, Kuwabara M, et al. Pineal arachnoid cyst demonstrated with magnetic resonance imaging. Canine Pract 2000;25:14–5.
13. Saito M, Olby NJ, Spaulding K. Identification of arachnoid cysts in the quadrigeminal cistern using ultrasonography. Vet Radiol Ultrasound 2001;42:435–9.
14. Vernau KM, LeCouteur RA, Sturges BK, et al. Intracranial intra-arachnoid cyst with intracystic hemorrhage in two dogs. Vet Radiol Ultrasound 2002;43:449–54.
15. Platt SR. What is your diagnosis? Intracranial intra-arachnoid cysts. J Small Anim Pract 2002;43:425.
16. Kitagawa M, Kanayama K, Sakai T. Quadrigeminal cisterna arachnoid cyst diagnosed by MRI in five dogs. Aust Vet J 2003;81:340–3.

17. Duque C, Parent J, Brisson B, et al. Intracranial arachnoid cysts: are they clinically significant? J Vet Intern Med 2005;19:772–4.
18. Dewey CW, Scrivani PV, Krotscheck U, et al. Intracranial arachnoid cysts in dogs. Compend Contin Educ Vet 2009;31:160–7 [quiz: 168].
19. Matiasek LA, Platt SR, Shaw S, et al. Clinical and magnetic resonance imaging characteristics of quadrigeminal cysts in dogs. J Vet Intern Med 2007;21:1021–6.
20. Dewey CW, Marino DJ, Bailey KS, et al. Craniotomy with cystoperitoneal shunting for treatment of intracranial arachnoid cysts in dogs [electronic resource]. Vet Surg 2007;36:416–22.
21. Ju-Won KIM, Dong-In J, Byeong-Teck K, et al. Unilateral facial paresis secondary to a suspected brainstem arachnoid cyst in a Maltese dog. J Vet Med Sci 2011; 73:459.
22. Rabiei K, Tisell M, Wikkelsø C, et al. Diverse arachnoid cyst morphology indicates different pathophysiological origins. Fluids Barriers CNS 2014;11:1–28.
23. Cincu R, Agrawal A, Eiras J. Review: intracranial arachnoid cysts: current concepts and treatment alternatives. Clin Neurol Neurosurg 2007;109:837–43.
24. Gosalakkal JA. Intracranial arachnoid cysts in children: a review of pathogenesis, clinical features, and management. Pediatr Neurol 2002;26:93–8.
25. Santamarta D, Aguas J, Ferrer E. The natural history of arachnoid cysts: endoscopic and cine-mode MRI evidence of a slit-valve mechanism. Minim Invasive Neurosurg 1995;38:133–7.
26. Yildiz H, Erdogan C, Yalcin R, et al. Evaluation of communication between intracranial arachnoid cysts and cisterns with phase-contrast cine MR imaging. AJNR Am J Neuroradiol 2005;26:145–51.
27. Wang C, Han G, You C, et al. Individual surgical treatment of intracranial arachnoid cyst in pediatric patients. Neurol India 2013;61:400–5.
28. Murthy JMK. Intracranial arachnoid cysts: epileptic seizures. Neurol India 2013; 61:343–4.
29. Chao W, Chuangxi L, Yunbiao X, et al. Surgical treatment of intracranial arachnoid cyst in adult patients. Neurol India 2013;61:60.
30. Mateo I. Diverticulum of the third ventricle and absence of the interthalamic adhesion in a dog. Can Vet J 2012;53:539–42.
31. Li L, Zhang Y, Li Y, et al. The clinical classification and treatment of middle cranial fossa arachnoid cysts in children. Clin Neurol Neurosurg 2013;115:411–8.
32. Khan IS, Sonig A, Thakur JD, et al. Surgical management of intracranial arachnoid cysts: clinical and radiological outcome. Turk Neurosurg 2013;23:138–43.
33. Yanamadala V, Lin N, Walcott BP, et al. Neuroradiology report: spontaneous regression of an epidermoid cyst of the cavernous sinus. J Clin Neurosci 2014; 21:1433–5.
34. De Decker S, Davies E, Benigni L, et al. Surgical treatment of an intracranial epidermoid cyst in a dog. Vet Surg 2012;41:766–71.
35. Steinberg T, Matiasek K, Brühschwein A, et al. Imaging diagnosis: intracranial epidermoid cyst in a Doberman pinscher. Vet Radiol Ultrasound 2007;48:250–3.
36. MacKillop E, Schatzberg SJ, De Lahunta A. Intracranial epidermoid cyst and syringohydromyelia in a dog. Vet Radiol Ultrasound 2006;47:339–44.
37. Platt SR, Graham J, Chrisman CL, et al. Canine intracranial epidermoid cyst. Vet Radiol Ultrasound 1999;40:454–8.
38. Kawaminami A, Tawaratani T, Nakazawa M, et al. A case of multiloculated, intracranial epidermoid cyst in a Beagle dog. Lab Anim 1991;25:226–7.
39. Klaus B. Epidermoide des IV. Ventrikels beim Hund. [Epidermoid neoplasms of the fourth ventricle in the dog]. Schweiz Arch Tierheilkd 1972;114:430–8 [in German].

40. Mawdesley-Thomas LE, Hague PH. An intra-cranial epidermoid cyst in a dog. Vet Rec 1970;87:133–4.
41. Spoor MS, Spagnoli ST, Burton EN, et al. What is your diagnosis? Cystic mass in the fourth ventricle of the brain of a dog. Vet Clin Pathol 2013;42:387–8.
42. Kornegay JN, Gorgacz EJ. Intracranial epidermoid cysts in three dogs. Vet Pathol 1982;19:646–50.
43. Raghunath A, Devi BI, Bhat DI, et al. Unusual complications of a benign tumour: our experience with midline posterior fossa epidermoids. Br J Neurosurg 2013; 27:69–73.
44. Tuchman A, Platt A, Winer J, et al. Peer-review report: endoscopic-assisted resection of intracranial epidermoid tumors. World Neurosurg 2014;82:450–4.
45. Nagasawa DT, Choy W, Spasic M, et al. An analysis of intracranial epidermoid tumors with malignant transformation: treatment and outcomes. Clin Neurol Neurosurg 2013;115:1071–8.
46. Yamakawa K, Shitara N, Genka S, et al. Clinical course and surgical prognosis of 33 cases of intracranial epidermoid tumors. Neurosurgery 1989;24:568–73.
47. Cherian A, Baheti NN, Easwar HV, et al. Recurrent meningitis due to epidermoid. J Pediatr Neurosci 2012;7:47–8.
48. O'Brien DP, Jergens A, Nelson S. Intracranial epidermoid (cholesteatoma) associated with aseptic suppurative meningoencephalitis in an aged dog. J Am Anim Hosp Assoc 1990;26:582–5.
49. Benigni L, Lamb CR. Comparison of fluid-attenuated inversion recovery and T2-weighted magnetic resonance images in dogs and cats with suspected brain disease. Vet Radiol Ultrasound 2005;46:287–92.
50. Nguyen JB, Ahktar N, Delgado PN, et al. Magnetic resonance imaging and proton magnetic resonance spectroscopy of intracranial epidermoid tumors. Crit Rev Comput Tomogr 2004;45:389–427.
51. Gopalakrishnan CV, Ansari KA, Nair S, et al. Long term outcome in surgically treated posterior fossa epidermoids. Clin Neurol Neurosurg 2014;117:93–9.
52. Targett MP, McInnes E, Dennis R. Magnetic resonance imaging of a medullary dermoid cyst with secondary hydrocephalus in a dog. Vet Radiol Ultrasound 1999;40:23–6.
53. Howard-Martin M, Bowles MH. Intracranial dermoid cyst in a dog. J Am Vet Med Assoc 1988;192:215–6.
54. Orakcioglu B, Halatsch ME, Fortunati M, et al. Intracranial dermoid cysts: variations of radiological and clinical features. Acta Neurochir 2008;150:1227–34.
55. Lynch JC, Aversa A, Pereira C, et al. Surgical strategy for intracranial dermoid and epidermoid tumors: an experience with 33 Patients. Surg Neurol Int 2014;5:163.
56. Schneider UC, Koch A, Stenzel W, et al. Intracranial, supratentorial dermoid cysts in paediatric patients: two cases and a review of the literature. Childs Nerv Syst 2012;28:185–90.
57. Markus H, Kendall BE. MRI of a dermoid cyst containing hair. Neuroradiology 1993;35:256–7.
58. Esquenazi Y, Kerr K, Bhattacharjee MB, et al. Traumatic rupture of an intracranial dermoid cyst: case report and literature review. Surg Neurol Int 2013;4:80.
59. Sood S, Gupta R. Susceptibility artifacts in ruptured intracranial dermoid cysts: a poorly understood but important phenomenon. Neuroradiol J 2014;27:677–84.
60. Brewer DM, Cerda-Gonzalez S, Dewey CW, et al. Diagnosis and surgical resection of a choroid plexus cyst in a dog. J Small Anim Pract 2010;51:169–72.
61. Galano HR, Platt SR, Neuwirth L, et al. Choroid plexus cyst in a dog. Vet Radiol Ultrasound 2002;43:349–52.

62. de Lara D, Ditzel Filho LFS, Muto J, et al. Endoscopic treatment of a third ventricle choroid plexus cyst. Neurosurg Focus 2013;34:Video 9.

63. Eboli P, Danielpour M. Acute obstructive hydrocephalus due to a large posterior third ventricle choroid plexus cyst. Pediatr Neurosurg 2011;47:292–4.

64. Jeon JH, Lee SW, Ko JK, et al. Neuroendoscopic removal of large choroid plexus cyst: a case report. J Korean Med Sci 2005;20:335–9.

65. Binning MJ, Couldwell WT. Case report: choroid plexus cyst development and growth following ventricular shunting. J Clin Neurosci 2008;15:79–81.

66. Hanbali F, Fuller GN, Leeds NE, et al. Choroid plexus cyst and chordoid glioma. Report of two cases. Neurosurg Focus 2001;10:E5.

Atlantoaxial Instability

Meghan C. Slanina, DVM

KEYWORDS

- Atlantoaxial instability • Atlantoaxial subluxation • Cervical myelopathy • Dog

KEY POINTS

- Atlantoaxial instability is a congenital condition affecting toy breed dogs; however, large breed dogs and cats can also be affected, and traumatic atlantoaxial instability can occur in dogs of any age or breed.
- Radiographic findings consistent with atlantoaxial subluxation include dorsal displacement of the axis into the vertebral canal, an increased distance between the arch of the atlas and the spinous process of the axis, and a lack of or conformational changes to the dens.
- Although surgical management is advocated for when there are neurologic deficits or patients are refractory to medical management, there is no clear consensus on the most successful surgical technique.

INTRODUCTION

Atlantoaxial subluxation was first reported in dogs in 1967.[1] Congenital atlantoaxial subluxation typically occurs in young, toy breed dogs with overrepresentation by Yorkshire Terriers, Pomeranians, Miniature and Toy Poodles, Chihuahuas, and Pekingese,[2–7] although larger breed dogs and cats can be affected.[8–15] Congenital abnormalities contributing to atlantoaxial joint instability include dens aplasia, hypoplasia, dorsal angulation or degeneration, and failure or absence of ligamentous support.[16–19] Other congenital abnormalities that may contribute to instability include incomplete ossification of the atlas[20,21] or block vertebrae.[22] Acquired atlantoaxial subluxation can occur in any age or breed dog secondary to a traumatic event.[18] Since the initial report of atlantoaxial instability, multiple reports were published to elucidate the underlying predisposing causes of joint instability and subluxation and to compare the various proposed treatment options.

ANATOMY

The atlantoaxial joint is unique to allow pivot motion in a longitudinal plane; therefore, the anatomy of the first 2 cervical vertebrae is modified significantly from the remainder

Disclosure Statement: The author has nothing to disclose.
Department of Clinical Sciences, Cornell University Hospital for Animals, College of Veterinary Medicine, Cornell University, 53 Dart Drive, Ithaca, NY 14853, USA
E-mail address: Mcs379@cornell.edu

of the vertebrae to facilitate this function. The atlas, or C1, is the first cervical vertebra and articulates with the occipital bone and the axis, or C2. Unlike the other cervical vertebrae, the atlas lacks a spinous process, has large transverse processes known as the wings of the atlas, and has a reduced vertebral body that forms a ventral arch.[23,24] The lateral portions of the atlas are called the *lateral masses* and they connect the ventral and dorsal arches. The ventral arch contains a depression called the fovea of the dens, which articulates with the dens of the axis. The atlanto-occipital joint forms from the articulation of the cranial articular fovea on the cranial aspect of the ventral arch of the atlas and the occipital condyles of the skull and predominantly facilitates vertical head movements.[23] The caudal articular fovea are located on the dorsal aspect of the body of the atlas and articulate with the modified articular processes of the axis. The joint formed between the atlas and axis facilitates rotary head movement.[23]

The axis is the longest vertebra and is distinguished by a prominent spinous process and a bony protuberance from the cranioventral aspect of the vertebra, known as the odontoid process or dens.[23] The dens lies in the fovea of the dens in the atlas and is held in place by the transverse ligament, which lies dorsal to the dens.[25] There is a separate area of ossification at the apical aspect of the dens called the *proatlas*, which is suspected to be a remnant vertebrae in mammals. The proatlas ossifies and then fuses with the dens at around 106 days postpartum. Before fusion or with incomplete ossification, the proatlas can be mistaken for a fracture of the dens.[23]

In addition to the transverse ligament, the apical ligament of the dens and the 2 alar ligaments help stabilize the atlantoaxial joint. The apical ligament of the dens attaches the center of the apex of the dens to the basioccipital bone. The paired alar ligaments originate on either side of the apical ligament on the dens and diverge laterally to attach medial to the occipital condyles.[25] The thin, loose joint capsule of the atlantoaxial joint and the dorsal atlantoaxial membrane, which extends between the arches of the atlas and axis, also assist with joint alignment.[25,26]

A cadaveric study was performed to evaluate the stabilizing function of the individual atlantoaxial ligaments in dogs.[26] The biomechanical evaluation was performed on a shear testing device that provided shear loading in a dorsoventral direction. A study by Reber and colleagues[26] showed that the greatest stabilizing force of the atlantoaxial ligaments were the alar ligaments. Their findings differed from what is found in people, with the transverse ligaments providing the most anterior stability.[26,27]

CLINICAL SIGNS

Instability of the atlantoaxial joint often leads to overflexion causing dorsal subluxation of the axis relative to the atlas and subsequent spinal cord trauma.[28] The degree of a patient's clinical signs range from neck pain to paralysis and correlate with the compressive and concussive injury to the spinal cord from subluxation. In the most severe cases, subluxation can result in respiratory paralysis and death.[1] Both an acute and insidious onset of neurologic signs have been reported with atlantoaxial instability.[1,16]

An atlantoaxial subluxation should be suspected in any young, toy breed dog that presents with signs of a C1 to C5 myelopathy. On neurologic examination, particular care should be taken to avoid manipulation of the neck, especially ventroflexion. From selected literature, the following distribution of neurologic statuses were noted on presentation[4,16,29–37]:

- Neck pain, some with a mild ataxia in 24.9% of cases (54 of 217)
- Ambulatory with a moderate to severe ataxia or paresis in 34.1% of cases (74 of 217)

- Nonambulatory paraparetic in 34.5% of cases (75 of 217)
- Tetraplegic in 6.5% of cases (14 of 217)

Differential diagnoses for a young dog with a C1 to C5 myelopathy include meningomyelitis, a vertebral fracture, discospondylitis, a spinal arachnoid diverticulum, intervertebral disc disease, and, less likely, neoplasia. Intervertebral disc extrusions are uncommon in dogs less than a year of age, unless they are associated with a traumatic event. Neoplasia is also uncommon in young patients, and spinal arachnoid diverticula are often not associated with severe neck pain.

DIAGNOSIS

The diagnosis of atlantoaxial instability can typically be made on survey radiographs; however, advanced diagnostic imaging such as computed tomography (CT) and MRI may provide additional information and facilitate surgical planning.

Radiographic findings consistent with atlantoaxial subluxation include dorsal displacement of the axis into the vertebral canal, an increased distance between the arch of the atlas and the spinous process of the axis, and hypoplasia, aplasia, or dorsal angulation of the dens[4,5,35] (**Fig. 1**). If a diagnosis cannot be made with a single lateral cervical radiograph, careful, gentle flexion of the dog's neck can provide additional diagnostic information. Ideally, fluoroscopy should be used to obtain images dynamically to prevent subluxation and avoid worsening of neurologic status, respiratory paralysis, or death.[35] Although a lateral radiograph is typically all that is required for diagnosis, a ventrodorsal or oblique radiograph can aid in evaluation of the dens. McLear and Saunders[38] evaluated the atlantoaxial joint in normal dogs undergoing myelography to assess normal range of motion. They found that a decrease in angle between the axis and the atlas was a better predictor of atlantoaxial instability than atlantoaxial overlap, with an angle of less than 162° correlating with instability.[28,38]

Myelography has been described for the use of diagnosing atlantoaxial instability, but it is not ideal given the risks associated with myelographic studies[39,40] and the availability of other advanced diagnostic imaging modalities, such as CT and MRI. CT is the best imaging modality to evaluate bony elements of the vertebral column and is useful in evaluation of the structure of the dens and for ruling out fractures of the dens or vertebrae[20,41,42] (**Fig. 2A, C**). CT imaging is also useful in providing

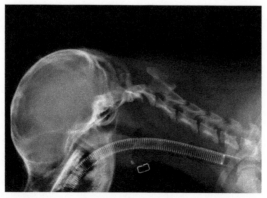

Fig. 1. Lateral radiograph of a 1-year-old Yorkshire Terrier shows subluxation of the atlantoaxial joint with displacement of the axis into the vertebral canal and an increased distance between the arch of the atlas and the spinous process of the axis.

information on bone corridor measurements and the development of 3-dimensional reconstructions for surgical planning.[43] Postoperative imaging via CT is beneficial to evaluate implant placement in relation to the spinal canal (see **Fig.** 2B, D; **Fig.** 3B).

MRI is an excellent modality for evaluating soft tissue structures; however, it is not as effective at bone evaluation as CT. It can be useful for evaluating intraparenchymal lesions that may be associated with atlantoaxial instability such as edema, hemorrhage, or syringomyelia, which may provide prognostic information, and for ruling out concurrent neurologic disease[44,45] (see **Fig.** 3A). In a human study, functional MRI is found to underestimate the degree of subluxation and should not be relied on as a sole diagnostic technique for ruling out this disease process.[36,46] A study by Middleton and colleagues[47] describes an MRI protocol for assessment of the ligaments and joint capsule at the level of the atlantoaxial joint; however, no studies correlate patient outcomes with ligamentous abnormalities at this time.

TREATMENT

The goal of medical treatment for atlantoaxial subluxation is the formation of fibrous tissue to stabilize the atlantoaxial joint and prevent further subluxation.[4] The goal of surgical treatment is reduction of the subluxation to resolve the compressive force and stabilization of the atlantoaxial joint to prevent further subluxation and contusion.[4]

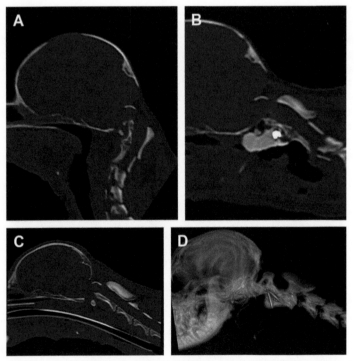

Fig. 2. Preoperative (*A*) and postoperative (*B*) midsagittal CT images of the atlantoaxial joint in a 10-month-old Chihuahua and a preoperative (*C*) midsagittal CT image and (*D*) postoperative 3-dimensional reconstruction of the atlantoaxial joint in a 6-month-old Chihuahua with atlantoaxial subluxation. (*A, C*) Severe and moderate subluxation, respectively, of the atlantoaxial joint. (*B, D*) Reduction of the luxations and stabilization with ventral screws and PMMA.

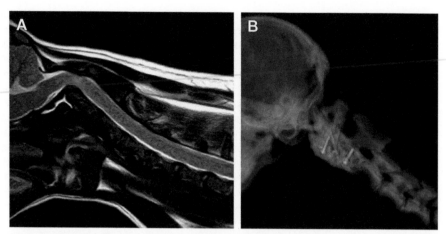

Fig. 3. Preoperative midsagittal MRI (*A*) and postoperative CT 3-dimensional (*B*) reconstruction of the atlantoaxial junction of a 9-month-old Yorkshire Terrier. (*A*) Note the increased distance between the arch of the atlas and spinous process of the axis, the dorsal deviation of the spinal cord, and the narrowing and hyperintensity in the spinal cord between C1 and C2. Postoperatively, note the reduction in distance between the arch of the atlas and spinous process of the axis.

Surgical treatment of atlantoaxial instability is typically advocated in patients with neurologic deficits or neck pain refractory to medical management, whereas medical management is typically reserved for dogs with only cervical hyperesthesia or minimal neurologic deficits, high-risk anesthetic candidates, those with minimal anatomic displacement, or when finances prevent surgical intervention.[4,35] Stabilization of the atlantoaxial joint provides many challenges, including the small size and immature bone of most patients, a small corridor for implant placement, and surgical proximity to vital structures; therefore, many different surgical approaches have been described to compare surgical efficacy and safety.[48]

Medical Management

Medical management consists of a cervical splint, pain management, and strict exercise restriction. Havig and colleagues[4] described the use of fiberglass ventral or dorsal splints that were incorporated into a soft padded bandage. The ventral splints extended from the mandible rostrally to the xiphoid caudally, whereas the dorsal splints extended from the caudal aspect of the bony orbit to the last thoracic vertebra. Dogs were rested with the cervical splint for a median of 8.5 weeks, and 62.5% (10 of 16) had a positive clinical outcome, which was defined as having a normal neurologic gait or being ambulatory with an ataxia or spasticity. Based on their results, the authors recommended consideration of medical management for patients with an acute history of neurologic signs, immature bones for which surgery may not provide adequate stabilization, or if owner finances did not allow for surgical stabilization.[4] Complications associated with a cervical splint were noted in 36.8% (7 of 19) of patients and included inadequate stabilization, moist dermatitis, skin ulceration, corneal ulceration, and decubital ulcers.[4]

Dorsal Surgical Procedures

The approach to a dorsal surgical procedure for atlantoaxial instability is technically less challenging and safer than a ventral procedure and provides good exposure;

however, a dorsal procedure does not provide access to the atlantoaxial joint for arthrodesis.[29,33] Because of the inability to provide atlantoaxial joint arthrodesis, dorsal procedures depend on implants to immobilize the joint until the formation of fibrous scar tissue.[49] Implants are placed in the cortical bone of C1 and C2, which is thin in most patients, and if the implants fail before the formation of fibrous tissue, neurologic signs may recur.[49]

Different types of dorsal procedures have been described in the literature to attach the dorsal arch of the atlas to the spinous process of the axis, including the use of a metal retractor, the nuchal ligament, orthopedic wire, or suture.[1,2,29,31,33,37,50–53] The placement of orthopedic wire or suture involves passage through the vertebral canal of the atlas, which can cause significant iatrogenic spinal cord damage and death.[33,36,37,50] Other dorsal procedures such as the Kishigami Atlantoaxial Tension Band, use of the nuchal ligament, use of loops of suture from the axis to the obliquus capitis cranialis muscle of the occipital bone, and dorsal pinning all help avoid the high-risk procedure of passing wire through the epidural space of the vertebral canal of the atlas.[31,33,34,52,53] Complications from dorsal procedures included breakage of suture, fracture of the axis, cardiorespiratory arrest, and loss of reduction.[29]

Ventral Surgical Procedures

A ventral surgical approach allows reduction of the luxation, access to the dens, and visualization of the atlantoaxial joint, which allows for curettage, bone grafts, and potentially eventual bony fusion; however, the approach involves dissection around vital structures including the carotid sheath, larynx, thyroid gland, and thyroid vasculature.[2,5,29,35,54] A ventral parasagittal approach has been described, which limited dissection, protected vital structures, and provided improved surgical site visualization.[35] Ventral procedures have been described for atlantoaxial stabilization through the use of plates, positively threaded profile pins, screws, and Kirschner wires; many of the procedures are performed with and without polymethylmethacrylate (PMMA).[2,29,30,32,35,37,45,54]

Before stabilization, reduction of the subluxation must be obtained. Forterre and colleagues[48] described a technique of using a small self-retracting gelpi placed in a C2 to C3 fenestration caudally and at the level of the atlanto-occipital junction cranially. This technique allowed for reduction of the joint without the loss of visualization that handheld instrumentation or vertebral screws entails. After reduction of the subluxation, removal of the articular cartilage and stabilization procedures are performed.

One of the benefits of a ventral surgical technique is the exposure of the atlantoaxial joint, allowing removal of the articular cartilage, placement of a bone graft, and arthrodesis providing stabilization long term.[30,49,54] Sorjonen and Shires[54] noted evidence of fibrous (3 of 10), cartilaginous (8 of 10), or bony union (4 of 10) on necropsy of the atlantoaxial joint in 10 of 12 dogs that were stabilized 6 weeks postoperatively. In procedures in which PMMA is used, it is difficult to assess arthrodesis radiographically because of poor visualization of the joint.[49] Although it has not been shown whether ankylosis of the atlantoaxial joint is necessary for long-term stabilization,[30,49] it is likely helpful.

Stabilization of the vertebral bodies is challenging in most patients; however, dogs with congenital atlantoaxial subluxations are typically small, toy breed dogs with immature bones, making the surgery even more demanding. Multiple procedures are reported, including the use of pins, locking plates, Kirschner wire, and vertebral body screws with and without PMMA.[2,29,30,32,35,37,45,54] Goals of many of the procedures are to maximize implant number and size to try to distribute the force of the stabilization, while keeping in mind the limited bone available for implant placement. A study involving CT determination of the bone corridor for transarticular screw placement in toy breed dogs showed a range of corridor diameters from 3 to 4.5 mm, with the narrowest aspect of the pathway reaching a maximum of 3.5 mm.[43] Given these measurements and the idea that maximizing screw diameter is important for minimizing screw pull out force, screws of 1.5 to 2 mm were recommended in toy breed dogs.[43]

PMMA is commonly used in ventral stabilization procedures that use pins, Kirschner wires, or screws, with a goal of preventing implant migration.[49] In one study, PMMA was used in 32.5% (13 of 40) of ventral procedures. Of the procedures for which PMMA was not used, wire migration was documented in 30% (8 of 27).[29] Complications of PMMA use include thermal injury, pressure necrosis, and infection.[29]

Complications from ventral procedures that necessitated an additional surgical procedure included implant migration, implant failure, or loss of reduction.[16,29] Additional complications were noted that did not require an additional surgery and included hemorrhage, aspiration pneumonia, laryngeal paralysis, coughing, gagging, dyspnea, Horner's syndrome, voice change, pin breakage, implant loosening or migration, fracture of the atlas or axis, tracheal injury or necrosis, esophageal stricture, and torticollis.[16,29,49]

PROGNOSIS

A study by Beaver and colleagues[29] comparing risk factors affecting the outcome of atlantoaxial stabilizing surgeries found comparable success rates for dorsal (88.9%) and ventral (85.3%) procedures; however, dogs were noted to have a higher incidence of postoperative neurologic deficits with dorsal procedures (44.4% ataxia, 11.1% cervical pain) compared with ventral procedures (19.4% ataxia, 9.7% cervical pain). In comparison, 62.5% of patients managed medically had a positive neurologic outcome.[4] Factors affecting a patient's outcome other than the type of surgical technique were evaluated. An acute onset of clinical signs was found to be a positive predictor of a successful neurologic outcome.[4,29] Age of onset of clinical signs was found to be moderately predictive of outcome in some studies,[29] although this finding did not emerge in all studies.[4,16] Severity of neurologic deficits at presentation has shown a mild correlation with outcome in some studies,[16,29] although other studies noted that many patients with the most significant neurologic deficits improved to normal neurologic examinations.[4,33,34,37] Postoperative atlantoaxial reduction and radiographic appearance of the dens did not correlate with outcome.[29]

Direct comparison of the outcomes of various studies is difficult because each study uses different criteria for successful outcomes and neurologic scoring systems. **Table 1** provides a comparison of outcomes from dorsal procedures, ventral procedures, and medical management from selected literature.[4,16,29–37] In this table, an excellent outcome is defined as a final neurologic grade of 4 or 5 (ambulatory with ataxia or ambulatory with a normal gait with or without neck pain, respectively),[32] a satisfactory outcome is defined as ambulatory with paresis, which included some animals with implant failure or secondary vertebral fracture that did not require a second surgery to correct the implant failure. If a second surgery was required, the first surgery was considered unsuccessful, and the second surgery was based on the original criteria. Animals lost to follow-up were not considered (see **Table 1**).

Plessas and Volk[6] presented an abstract of a systematic review of the 336 published cases from 1967 to 2013. They found that 84.5% (284 of 336) dogs underwent surgery with 70.8% (201 of 284) of those dogs receiving a ventral procedure and 29.2% (83 of 284) receiving a dorsal procedure. A successful outcome was reported

Table 1
Comparison of outcomes in medically and surgically managed atlantoaxial subluxation cases in selected literature

| Author | Medical Management | | |
	Excellent[a]	Satisfactory[b]	Death or Euthanasia[c]
Havig et al,[4] 2005	62.5% (10/16)	62.5% (10/16)	37.5% (6/16)
	Dorsal Surgical		
Pujol et al,[33] 2010	75% (6/8)	75% (6/8)	25% (2/8)
Jeffery,[31] 1996	100% (1/1)	100% (1/1)	0% (0/1)
Sánchez-Masian et al,[34] 2004[d]	68.8% (11/16)	68.8% (11/16)	6.3% (1/16)
Dickomeit et al,[30] 2011	100% (3/3)	100% (3/3)	0% (0/3)
Thomas et al,[37] 1991[d]	37.5% (3/8)	62.5% (5/8)	14.3% (1/7)
Beaver et al,[29] 2000[d]	75% (9/12)	75% (9/12)	8.3% (1/12)
Total	68.8% (33/48)	72.9% (35/48)	10.1% (5/47)
	Ventral Surgical		
Sánchez-Masian et al,[34] 2014[d]	100% (2/2)	100% (2/2)	0% (0/2)
Shores & Tepper,[35] 2007	100% (5/5)	100% (5/5)	0% (0/5)
Platt et al,[32] 2004	63.2% (12/19)	84.2% (16/19)	15.8% (3/19)
Aikawa et al,[16] 2013	81.6% (40/49)	93.9% (46/49)	4.1% (2/49)
Thomas et al,[37] 1991[d]	50% (10/20)	50% (10/20)	38.9% (7/18)
Beaver et al,[29] 2000[d]	77.5% (31/40)	77.5% (31/40)	12.5% (5/40)
Total	74.1% (100/135)	81.5% (110/135)	12.8% (17/133)

[a] Excellent—neurologic score of 4 (ambulatory with ataxia) or 5 (normal ± neck pain); out of number of surgical procedures.
[b] Satisfactory—neurologic score of 3 (ambulatory with paresis) or higher; out of number of surgical procedures.
[c] Death or euthanasia—Secondary to clinical signs of atlantoaxial subluxation or surgical complications; out of number of patients that received surgery.
[d] Represents studies where more than one procedure was performed on some subjects.

in 82.6% (166 of 201) of ventral procedures and 65.1% (54 of 83) of dorsal procedures. Medical management was pursued in 11.6% (39 of 336) of cases with 71.8% (28 of 39) of dogs having a positive outcome as defined by final neurologic scores of 4 or 5 (ambulatory with an ataxia and ambulatory with no neurologic deficits, respectively). The perioperative fatality rate was 5% with ventral procedures and 8% with dorsal procedures.[6]

Both acute and chronic spinal cord injuries can result in pathologic changes such as demyelination, axonal degeneration, gliosis, or malacia, which may be permanent and nonresponsive to surgical management.[4,29,33,55] Continued instability or concurrent neurologic disease may also be responsible for progressive or unrelenting neurologic signs in those patients that do not improve with treatment.[4,29]

SUMMARY

Atlantoaxial instability is a congenital neurologic condition predominantly affecting toy breed dogs. Neurologic signs of a cranial cervical myelopathy typically present at a young age and can range from cervical pain to paralysis. Diagnosis is based on survey radiographs, although advanced diagnostic imaging can facilitate surgical planning, allow evaluation of spinal cord parenchyma, and rule out concurrent neurologic conditions. Treatment options consist of medical or surgical management, with surgical management being preferable in patients with neurologic deficits or those with unresolved cervical pain despite medical management. The prognosis for surgery is usually favorable. Prognostic indicators of a positive outcome include an acute onset of neurologic signs and a younger age at presentation.

REFERENCES

1. Geary J, Oliver J, Hoerlein BF. Atlanto axial subluxation in the canine. J Small Anim Pract 1967;8:577–82.
2. Denny HR, Gibbs C, Waterman A. Atlantoaxial subluxation in the dog: a review of thirty cases and evaluation of treatment by lag screw fixation. J Small Anim Pract 1988;29:37–47.
3. Dewey CW, da Costa RC. Myelopathies: disorders of the spinal cord. In: Dewey CW, da Costa RC, editors. Practical guide to canine and feline neurology. 3rd edition. Ames (IA): Wiley-Blackwell; 2016. p. 329–405.
4. Havig ME, Cornell KK, Hawthorne JC, et al. Evaluation of nonsurgical treatment of atlantoaxial subluxation in dogs: 19 cases (1992-2001). J Am Vet Med Assoc 2005;227:257–62.
5. McCarthy RJ, Lewis DD, Hosgood G. Atlantoaxial subluxation in dogs. Compend Contin Educ Pract Vet 1995;17:215–27.
6. Plessas IN, Volk HA. Signalment, clinical signs and treatment of altantoaxial subluxation in dogs: a systematic review of 336 published cases from 1967 to 2013. J Vet Intern Med 2014;28:944–75.
7. Wheeler SJ, Sharp NJH. Atlantoaxial subluxation. In: Wheeler SJ, Sharp NJH, editors. Small animal spinal disorders. Diagnosis and surgery. London: Mosby-Wolfe; 1994. p. 109–21.
8. Huibregtse BA, Smith CW, Fagin BD. Atlantoaxial luxation in a doberman pinscher. Canine Practice 1992;17:7–10.
9. Hurov L. Congenital atlantoaxial malformation and acute subluxation in a mature basset hound – surgical treatment by wire stabilization. J Am Anim Hosp Assoc 1979;15:177–80.
10. Jaggy A, Hutto VL, Roberts RE, et al. Occipitoatlantoaxial malformation with atlantoaxial subluxation in a cat. J Small Anim Pract 1991;32:366–72.
11. Shelton SB, Bellah J, Chrisman C, et al. Hypoplasia of the odontoid process and secondary atlantoaxial luxation in a Siamese cat. Progr Vet Neurol 1991;2:209–11.
12. Stigen Ø, Aleksandersen M, Sørby R, et al. Acute non-ambulatory tetraparesis with absence of the dens in two large breed dogs: case reports with a radiographic study of relatives. Acta Vet Scand 2013;55:31.
13. Thomson MJ, Read RA. Surgical stabilization of the atlantoaxial joint in a cat. Vet Comp Orthop Traumatol 1996;9:36–9.
14. Watson AG, Hall MA, de Lahunta A. Congenital occipitoatlantoaxial malformation in a cat. Compend Contin Educ Pract Vet 1985;7:245–53.
15. Wheeler SJ. Atlantoaxial subluxation with absence of the dens in a rottweiler. J Small Anim Pract 1992;33:90–3.
16. Aikawa T, Shibata M, Fujita H. Modified ventral stabilization using positively threaded profile pins and polymethylmethacrylate for atlantoaxial instability in 49 dogs. Vet Surg 2013;42:683–92.
17. Ladds P, Guffy M, Blauch B, et al. Congenital odontoid process separation in two dogs. J Small Anim Pract 1971;12:463–71.

18. Oliver JE, Lewis RE. Lesions of the atlas and axis in dogs. J Am Anim Hosp Assoc 1973;9:304–13.
19. Watson AG, de Lahunta A. Atlantoaxial subluxation and absence of transverse ligament of the atlas in a dog. J Am Vet Med Assoc 1989;195:235–7.
20. Parry AT, Upjohn MM, Schleg K, et al. Computed tomography variations in morphology of the canine atlas in dogs with and without atlantoaxial subluxation. Vet Radiol Ultrasound 2010;52:596–600.
21. Warren-Smith CM, Kneissl S, Benigni L, et al. Incomplete ossification of the atlas in dogs with cervical signs. Vet Radiol Ultrasound 2009;50:635–8.
22. Lin JL, Coolman BR. Atlantoaxial subluxation in two dogs with cervical block vertebrae. J Am Anim Hosp Assoc 2009;45:305–10.
23. Evans HE, de Lahunta A. The skeleton. In: Evans HE, de Lahunta A, editors. Miller's anatomy of the dog. 4th edition. Philadelphia: WB Saunders; 2013. p. 80–157.
24. Dyce KM, Sack WO, Wensing CJG. The locomotor apparatus. In: Textbook of veterinary anatomy. 3rd edition. Philadelphia: WB Saunders; 1996. p. 35–8.
25. Evans HE, de Lahunta A. Arthrology. In: Evans HE, de Lahunta A, editors. Miller's anatomy of the dog. 4th edition. Philadelphia: WB Saunders; 2013. p. 158–85.
26. Reber K, Bürki A, Vizcaino Reves N, et al. Biomechanical evaluation of the stabilizing function of the atlantoaxial ligaments under shear loading: a canine cadaveric study. Vet Surg 2013;42:918–23.
27. Fielding JW, Van B, Cocran G, et al. Tears of the transverse ligament of the atlas. J Bone Joint Surg 1974;56A:1683–91.
28. Platt SR, da Costa RC. Cervical spine. In: Tobias KM, Johnston SA, editors. Veterinary surgery. St Louis (MO): Elsevier/Saunders; 2012. p. 410–48.
29. Beaver DP, Ellison GW, Lewis DD, et al. Risk factors affecting the outcome of surgery for atlantoaxial subluxation in dogs: 46 cases (1978-1998). J Am Vet Med Assoc 2000;216:1104–9.
30. Dickomeit M, Alves L, Pekarkova M, et al. Use of a 1.5 mm butterfly locking plate for stabilization of atlantoaxial pathology in three toy breed dogs. Vet Comp Orthop Traumatol 2011;24:246–51.
31. Jeffery ND. Dorsal cross pinning of the atlantoaxial joint: new surgical technique for atlantoaxial subluxation. J Small Anim Pract 1996;37:26–9.
32. Platt SR, Chambers JN, Cross A. A modified ventral fixation for surgical management of atlantoaxial subluxation in 19 dogs. Vet Surg 2004;33:349–54.
33. Pujol E, Bouvy B, Omaña M, et al. Use of the Kishigami atlantoaxial tension band in eight toy breed dogs with atlantoaxial subluxation. Vet Surg 2010; 39:35–42.
34. Sánchez-Masian D, Luján-Feliu-Pascual A, Font C, et al. Dorsal stabilization of atlantoaxial subluxation using non-absorbable sutures in toy breed dogs. Vet Comp Orthop Traumatol 2014;27:62–7.
35. Shores A, Tepper LC. A modified ventral approach to the atlantoaxial junction in the dog. Vet Surg 2007;36:765–70.
36. Stalin C, Gutierrez-Quintana R, Faller K, et al. A review of canine atlantoaxial joint subluxation. Vet Comp Orthop Traumatol 2015;28:1–8.
37. Thomas WB, Sorjonen DC, Simpson ST. Surgical management of atlantoaxial subluxation in 23 dogs. Vet Surg 1991;20:409–12.
38. McLear RC, Saunders HM. Atlantoaxial mobility in the dog. Vet Radiol Ultrasound 2000;41:558.
39. Barone G, Ziemer LS, Shofer FS, et al. Risk factors associated with development of seizures after use of iohexol for myelography in dogs: 182 cases (1998). J Am Vet Med Assoc 2002;220:1499–502.

40. Lewis DD, Hosgood G. Complications associated with the use of iohexol for mye-lography of the cervical vertebral column in dogs: 66 cases (1988-1990). J Am Vet Med Assoc 1992;200:1381–4.
41. Bahr A. The vertebrae. In: Thrall DE, editor. Textbook of veterinary diagnostic imaging. 5th edition. St Louis (MO): Elsevier; 2007. p. 179–93.
42. Drees R, Dennison SE, Keuler NS, et al. Computed tomographic imaging protocol for the canine cervical and lumbar spine. Vet Radiol Ultrasound 2009;50:74–9.
43. Vizcaíno Revés N, Stahl C, Stoffel M, et al. CT scan based determination of optimal bone corridor for atlantoaxial ventral screw fixation in miniature breed dogs. Vet Surg 2013;42:819–24.
44. Kent M, Eagleson JS, Neravanda D, et al. Intraaxial spinal cord hemorrhage sec-ondary to atlantoaxial subluxation in a dog. J Am Anim Hosp Assoc 2010;46:132–7.
45. Sanders SG, Bagley RS, Silver GM, et al. Outcomes and complications associ-ated with ventral screws, pins and polymethyl methacrylate for atlantoaxial insta-bility in 12 dogs. J Am Anim Hosp Assoc 2004;40:204–10.
46. Laiho K, Soini I, Kautiainen H, et al. Can we rely on magnetic resonance imaging when evaluating unstable atlantoaxial subluxation? Ann Rheum Dis 2003;62:254–6.
47. Middleton G, Hillman DJ, Trichel J, et al. Magnetic resonance imaging of the liga-mentous structures of the occipitoatlantoaxial region in the dog. Vet Radiol Ultra-sound 2012;53:545–51.
48. Forterre F, Vizcaino Revés N, Stahl C, et al. An indirect reduction technique for ventral stabilization of atlantoxial instability in miniature breed dogs. Vet Comp Orthop Traumatol 2012;25:332–6.
49. Schulz KS, Waldron DR, Fahie M. Application of ventral pins and polymethylme-thacrylate for the management of atlantoaxial instability: results in nine dogs. Vet Surg 1997;26:317–25.
50. Chambers JN, Betts CW, Oliver JE. The use of non-metallic suture material for stabilization of atlantoaxial subluxation. J Am Anim Hosp Assoc 1977;13:602–4.
51. Johnson P, Beltran E, Dennis R, et al. Magnetic resonance imaging characteris-tics of suspected vertebral instability association with fracture of subluxation in eleven dogs. Vet Radiol Ultrasound 2012;53:552–9.
52. Kishigami M. Application of an atlantoaxial retractor for atlantoaxial subluxation in the cat and dog. J Am Anim Hosp Assoc 1984;20:413–9.
53. LeCouteur RA, McKeown D, Johnson J, et al. Stabilization of atlantoaxial sublux-ation in the dog, using the nuchal ligament. J Am Vet Med Assoc 1980;177:1011–7.
54. Sorjonen DC, Shires PK. Atlantoaxial instability: a ventral surgical technique for decompression, fixation and fusion. Vet Surg 1981;1:22–9.
55. Griffiths IR, Burns N, Crawford AR. Early vascular changes in the spinal grey matter following impact injury. Acta Neuropathol 1978;35:135–46.

Cystic Abnormalities of the Spinal Cord and Vertebral Column

Ronaldo C. da Costa, DMV, MSc, PhD*, Laurie B. Cook, DVM

KEYWORDS

- Synovial cyst • Arachnoid diverticulum • Cysts • Dilated subarachnoid space

KEY POINTS

- Cystic lesions of the vertebral column and spinal cord are an important differential diagnosis in dogs with signs of spinal cord disease.
- Synovial cysts are commonly associated with degenerative joint disease and commonly affect the cervical and lumbosacral regions.
- Arachnoid diverticulum (previously known as cysts) is common in the cervical region of large breed dogs and thoracolumbar region of small breed dogs.
- This article reviews the causes, diagnosis, and treatment of these and other, less common, cystic lesions.

INTRODUCTION

Cystic lesions of the vertebral column and spinal cord are being recognized more commonly in veterinary patients concomitant with more frequent access to improved imaging such as MRI and computed tomographic (CT) myelography. These lesions may cause clinical signs, including paresis, ataxia, radiculopathy, and pain, whereas others may occur as incidental findings. Clinical assessment of a patient suspected of having a cystic spinal lesion includes physical and neurologic examination to localize the presence of a neurologic lesion. Imaging findings may then help to confirm the presence of a cystic lesion and the most likely differential diagnoses. Some cystic lesions may occur in conjunction with other congenital or acquired disease processes. The clinician must determine which is the most significant abnormality in such cases. With increased recognition of these conditions in veterinary patients, medical or surgical interventions can be tailored to the patient. This article describes the main cystic

The authors have nothing to disclose.
Department of Veterinary Clinical Sciences, College of Veterinary Medicine, The Ohio State University, Columbus, OH 43210-1089, USA
* Corresponding author.
E-mail address: dacosta.6@osu.edu

Vet Clin Small Anim 46 (2016) 277–293
http://dx.doi.org/10.1016/j.cvsm.2015.10.010
vetsmall.theclinics.com

lesions in the vertebral column and spinal cord in veterinary patients and reviews the current literature and controversies surrounding some of these diagnoses.

EXTRADURAL SYNOVIAL CYSTS
Cause and Pathogenesis

Extradural synovial and extradural intraspinal cysts arise from periarticular joint tissue. They can be divided into 2 cyst types: synovial and ganglion. Synovial cysts have a synovial lining containing fluid and ganglion cysts contain myxoid material with no specific lining. These are pathologic differences that may reflect different stages of the same disease.[1] Some investigators have suggested a synovial cyst may develop into a ganglion cyst or a ganglion cyst may develop a synovial lining over time.[2] Clinically, this distinction seems irrelevant, and, because both types of cysts occur in close proximity with the intervertebral joints, the term juxtafacet cysts has been coined to include both cysts.[1–3] The pathophysiology of development of these cysts is not well established. It is thought that degeneration of the zygapophyseal joint (osteoarthritic changes) and increased motion at the joint causes protrusion of the synovial membrane through defects of the joint capsule. Protrusion of the synovial membrane will cause the formation of a para-articular cavity filled with synovial fluid, which leads to extradural compression (**Fig. 1**).[1,2] Other proposed mechanisms are proliferation of pluripotent mesenchymal cells, myxoid degeneration with cyst formation in collagen tissue, and increased production of hyaluronic acid by fibroblasts.[2] Spinal instability or excessive mobility has been suggested as a cause, which is supported in that the 2 most common locations for synovial cyst formation are the lumbosacral region and the caudal cervical region, the latter of which is the area of greatest cervical mobility.[1,4] In humans, vertebral column instability is thought to play a factor in synovial cyst development because they occur with high frequency at the lumbar vertebra (L) 4 to L5 level, which is the most mobile region of the vertebral column, and because of their frequent association with osteoarthritis (40.5%), spondylolisthesis (43.3%), and disc degeneration (13.2%).[5] Synovial cysts in dogs are commonly associated with cervical spondylomyelopathy and the distribution of lesions mirrors the distribution of osseous compressions of the cervical spinal cord.[1,2,6] The precise

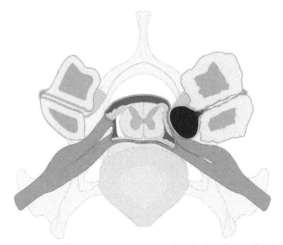

Fig. 1. A synovial cyst extending from degenerated articular facets (articular processes) in the cervical vertebral column. (*Courtesy of* The Ohio State University, Columbus, OH, 2016; with permission.)

mechanism is not known but all dogs with synovial cysts and cervical spondylomyel-opathy have concurrent vertebral column degenerative diseases that likely contribute to different stressors on the vertebral column.[1] There are 2 isolated reports of synovial cysts occurring with cranial cervical malformations. The first was a case in a Chihuahua with a synovial cyst arising from the atlantoaxial articulation.[7] The other was a case in a Cavalier King Charles spaniel with bilateral synovial cysts associated with degenerative arthropathy of the cervical vertebra (C) 2 to C3 articular facets.[8] The mechanism of formation in thoracolumbar and lumbosacral extradural synovial cysts is also not clear; however, increased mechanical stresses and instability have been proposed.[1,9] Some of the affected dogs with lumbosacral cysts had transitional verte-brae and this may be a risk factor.[10,11]

Clinical Findings

The clinical signs of synovial cysts reflect their location in the vertebral column, with the 2 most frequent locations being the lumbosacral and cervical regions (**Figs. 2 and 3**). Clinical signs of cervical cysts are those of a cervical myelopathy with propri-oceptive ataxia and tetraparesis, whereas pelvic limb lameness or weakness, with or without hyperesthesia on palpation, can be appreciated with lumbosacral cysts.[2,10,11] There are reports of synovial cyst formation in the thoracolumbar spine of large breed dogs that presented with signs of thoracolumbar myelopathy. These all occurred be-tween thoracic vertebra (T) 13 and L4.[2,11–13]

Diagnosis

Most dogs reported with lumbosacral or caudal lumbar synovial cysts were large breed, middle-aged, or older dogs (median age 8 years).[1] Cervical synovial cysts are relatively common in association with the osseous form of cervical spondylomyel-opathy in young, giant breed dogs.[2,6,14,15] Two studies that investigated the MRI appearance of cervical spondylomyelopathy indicated that synovial cysts occur in 20% of affected dogs.[14,15]

Diagnosis of synovial cysts is best accomplished with MRI (see **Figs. 2** and **3**). MRI reveals the cysts as well-circumscribed extradural masses on 1 or both sides of the vertebral canal associated with the articular processes. They are hyperintense on T2-weighted images, with variable low-signal intensity on T1-weighted images. The T1 signal can vary depending on the protein concentration of the fluid or the presence of hemorrhage.[5,6,10,11] In humans, MRI is reported to have a sensitivity of 90% for the diagnosis of extradural synovial cysts, compared with 70% with CT.[5] Both soft tissue and bone windows have to be used to increase accuracy of CT to detect these cysts

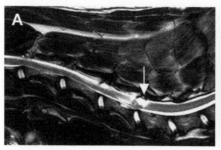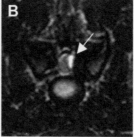

Fig. 2. Synovial cyst in the cervical region of a Rottweiler dog with cervical spondylomyel-opathy. (*A*) Sagittal and (*B*) transverse T2-weighted MRI showing the synovial cyst at C5-6 (*arrows*). Note the enlarged articular processes associated with the cyst on (*B*).

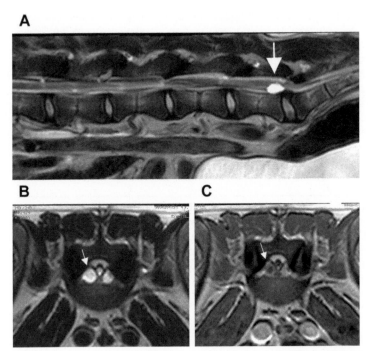

Fig. 3. Synovial cysts in the lumbosacral region of a German shepherd dog. (*A*) Sagittal T2-weighted image showing the cyst (*arrow*). (*B*) Transverse T2-weighted and (*C*) transverse T1-weighted images after administration of intravenous contrast showing the cysts (*arrows*).

and sometimes myelography has to be used in conjunction with CT (**Fig. 4**). Radiographic changes are nonspecific and will only indicate degenerative joint disease in the articular processes of affected sites.[2] Myelographic changes may be suggestive of synovial cysts but are not diagnostic. Changes in the lateral projection indicate dorsal extradural compression. In the ventrodorsal view, unilateral or bilateral axial compression is appreciated; this is due to proliferation of articular process and extension of soft tissue medially from the articular processes into the vertebral canal representing proliferative synovial tissue.[2] Cerebrospinal fluid (CSF) typically reveals

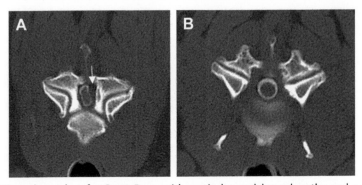

Fig. 4. CT myelography of a Great Dane with cervical spondylomyelopathy and a synovial cyst. (*A*) Note the thickened articular process and the cyst compressing the spinal cord (*arrow*) at C5-6. (*B*) Transverse image at C4-5 showing a normal region for comparison.

albuminocytologic dissociation but mild mononuclear pleocytosis may also be seen.[1,2]

Treatment

Treatment of these cysts is typically surgical. It is often done at the same time as the decompressive surgery (dorsal laminectomy) for cervical spondylomyelopathy or degenerative lumbosacral stenosis. In humans, however, many of these cysts are incidental findings.[3] Nonsurgical treatment in humans includes bed rest, physiotherapy, analgesics, and corticosteroid injections. Success rates with conservative treatment in humans ranges from 33% to 57%.[3] The same may be true for dogs. Therefore, attempting medical management with activity restriction and anti-inflammatory medications is recommended initially. Surgical treatment seems to produce better outcomes in humans when medical therapy fails, with good to excellent long-term outcomes reported as high as 83%.[5] All reported cases of surgical treatment of synovial cysts in dogs had positive outcomes.[1,2,6,9–13] Recurrence rates of synovial cyst formation in dogs is not known but is rarely reported in humans after surgical removal.[5]

SPINAL ARACHNOID DIVERTICULA (CYSTS)
Causes and Pathogenesis

Spinal arachnoid diverticula (SAD) are focal fluid-filled dilations of the subarachnoid space, which can lead to a progressive, compressive myelopathy. These diverticula were previously called arachnoid cysts but this is a misnomer because they are not true cysts.[1,16,17] The term cyst refers to a closed epithelial lined cavity filled with fluid, air, or other soft tissue substance.[1] Arachnoid diverticula are not epithelial-lined cavities. Therefore, the terms diverticula and pseudocyst are often used. They have also been called intra-arachnoid or subarachnoid cysts, meningeal cysts, and leptomeningeal cysts.[18–20] There are well-described classification schemes in human medicine and Lowrie and colleagues[1] recently proposed a classification scheme for veterinary patients.

Three types of meningeal cysts exist in human patients. Type 1 meningeal cysts are extradural cysts that do not involve the spinal nerves. Type 1a result from herniation of arachnoid membrane through a congenital or acquired dural defect and occur most commonly in adolescents. Type 1b are technically considered meningoceles but are attached by a pedicle to the dural sac, causing a dural diverticulum. These are most commonly seen in the sacral region in middle-age to elderly patients. Type 1 cysts have not been reported in domestic animals. Type 2 meningeal cysts are extradural cysts involving the spinal nerves and are an out-pouching of the perineurium surrounding the spinal nerve. These are also called Tarlov cysts. Type 3 meningeal cysts are intradural arachnoid diverticula (**Fig. 5**). These are not true cysts because they contain no epithelial lining and seem to communicate freely with the subarachnoid space. This form is most commonly recognized in canine patients as SAD.

The cause of these cysts is not fully understood. It seems that a congenital cause is likely in the cases seen in young dogs. Rarely, they have been reported in litter mates, supporting a genetic predisposition in some dogs.[21] A recent report indicated a genetic predisposition in pugs.[16] Pathophysiology is uncertain but they likely arise from a developmental abnormality of the arachnoid architecture.[18,19,22] It is thought that splitting of the arachnoid membrane occurs at some point during embryonic development. Expansion of this pocket can occur throughout life, resulting in a progressive spinal cord compression. A CSF-flow disturbance is thought to result in a

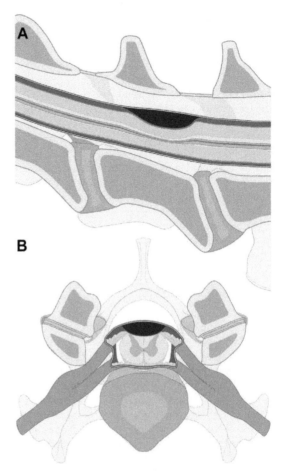

Fig. 5. Arachnoid diverticulum: (*A*) sagittal and (*B*) transverse views. The arachnoid layer separates forming the cystic-like structure and causes extradural compression of the spinal cord. (*Courtesy of* The Ohio State University, Columbus, OH, 2016; with permission.)

functional one-way valve into the pocket that allows CSF to flow in but not be released in response to changes in CSF pressure.[1,23,24]

Acquired SAD may also occur secondary to other disease processes. A large, recent case series indicated that 21.3% of dogs had concurrent diseases in close proximity with the diverticula, which might have influenced its development.[25] In particular, pug dogs (33.3%) and French bulldogs (61.5%) had high rates of concurrent disease, including intervertebral disc extrusion or protrusion, concurrent vertebral malformation, or previous surgery for intervertebral disc extrusion (**Fig. 6**).[25] They may occur secondary to chronic spinal cord compression from intervertebral disc disease,[18,26–28] spinal trauma,[20,27,29] and inflammatory spinal cord disease.[1,30] These diverticula may result from scarring, inflammation, or fibrin accumulation secondary to the underlying spinal disease. The association is inferred based on proximity to the other underlying disease.[1]

Two recent studies reviewed 215 cases of SAD.[1,25] These studies revealed that approximately 55% of these diverticula occur in the cervical region, whereas 45% are seen in the thoracolumbar region. The most common specific sites were

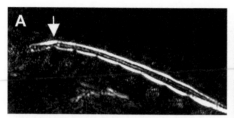
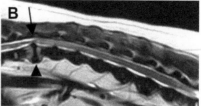

Fig. 6. MRI of a pug with a thoracolumbar arachnoid diverticulum secondary to spinal cord compression from an intervertebral disc protrusion. (*A*) Sagittal half-fourier acquisition single-shot turbo spin-echo pulse sequence (HASTE) image showing the diverticulum (*arrow*). (*B*) Sagittal T2-weighted image demonstrating the diverticulum (*arrow*) and disc protrusion (*arrowhead*).

C2 and C3, C5, and C6, and T9 to T13.[20,25,28,31] Large breed dogs have a predilection for cervical diverticula, with Rottweilers being overrepresented. It has been suggested that young, heavier dogs with large heads may be predisposed to cervical SAD.[5,19,20] Small breed dogs have a tendency to have thoracolumbar diverticula.[1,25] Males are overrepresented.[1,25] In humans, two-thirds of SAD patients are male and a possible hormonal influence on SAD formation has been suggested.[32] Progesterone receptors have been identified in the lining of intracranial arachnoid cysts in humans.[33,34] In addition, CSF volume has been shown to be influenced by hormonal fluctuations.[35] The effect of hormonal influences on development of SAD in dogs is not known and may warrant further investigation. Approximately 83% to 90% of the diverticula seem to be located in the dorsal aspect of the spinal cord (see **Figs. 5** and **6**), 6.4% to 8% in the ventral region, and the remainder in the lateral or circumferential regions.[1,25]

Clinical Signs

Clinical signs reflect the location of the myelopathy. This disease is primarily characterized by proprioceptive ataxia with various degrees of tetraparesis or paraparesis, with variable degrees of spinal-associated hyperpathia. Because SAD have a tendency to compress the dorsolateral spinal cord, compression of the ascending proprioceptive pathways and spinocerebellar tracts is often involved. As a result, a common feature is a severe spastic gait in the thoracic limbs, giving the appearance of pseudohypermetria.[36] Some dogs with cervical diverticulum will display more severe signs in the thoracic limbs, suggesting an intramedullary lesion. Spinal hyperpathia is not a consistent sign but has been reported in 18.9% of dogs in a large case series. Some of these subjects likely had underlying concurrent vertebral or spinal cord diseases that could have been responsible for the hyperpathia.[25] However, other previous case reports do describe variable spinal-associated hyperpathia in dogs with SAD.[9,18,23,26] Urinary and fecal incontinence have been reported in up to 8% of dogs, primarily with thoracolumbar diverticula.[25,30] The incidence of upper motor neuron fecal incontinence is more common with SAD than with other spinal cord disorders. It is suggested that impairment of dorsal sensory pathways in the spinal cord is responsible for this sign.[25,30]

Diagnosis

Three breeds are overrepresented: Rottweilers, pugs, and French bulldogs.[25] Median age at presentation in 2 large case series was 27 months (range 4–144 months)[1] and 36 months (mean 46 months).[25] Pugs were significantly older than other dog breeds at presentation (median age 59 months). This may reflect their tendency to develop SAD secondary to other spinal diseases such as intervertebral disc disease.[1,25] The Dogue de Bordeaux had a lower age at onset (median 11 months) than other breeds.[25] Clinical signs were present for a median of 4 months (range, 2 weeks–48 months).[25] Overall, a male predisposition is clear, with a male to female ratio ranging between 2 to 1 and 3 to 1 in the larger case series.

Myelography, CT myelography, or MRI is required to diagnose this disorder (**Fig. 7**). Myelography and postmyelographic CT demonstrate these diverticula as contrast-filled tear-drop shaped expansions of the subarachnoid space.[1,18] Imaging studies may also reveal a block of the subarachnoid contrast column without filling of the subarachnoid diverticula. This may be due to a one-way valve that allows CSF flow periodically only with fluctuations in CSF pressure. Alternatively, contrast medium may only be able to enter from 1 direction because of its cranial or caudal opening.[1] Delayed imaging, 12 to 24 hours following myelography, has been looked at in humans to allow more time for contrast to flow into the SAD.[37] Cerebellomedullary cistern injection of myelographic contrast may enhance filling of cervical SAD better than lumbar injection but may artifactually collapse the spinal cord caudal to the diverticulum, leading clinicians to believe the diverticulum is further caudal than it truly is.[38] MRI is generally considered the imaging modality of choice to evaluate these diverticula because it also allows assessment of the spinal cord parenchyma and detection of comorbidities, such as syringomyelia. SAD are typically hyperintense on T2-weighted sequences, and isointense to hypointense on T1-weighted sequences (**Fig. 8**). Most are hypointense on fluid-attenuated inversion recovery (FLAIR) sequences.[25] In some cases, when the diverticulum does not have the typical appearance, CT myelography may depict it more clearly (**Fig. 9**). It is helpful to use MR myelogram sequences (half-fourier acquisition single-shot turbo spin-echo pulse sequence [HASTE]) to facilitate visualization of the diverticulum.[39] This sequence gives more than a 2-fold increase in SAD identification compared with T2-weighted sequence alone (**Figs. 6** and **10**). The addition of this sequence decreased false negatives from 75% to 47%; therefore, some SAD may still go undetected.[39] Despite the strengths of MRI, differentiating between spinal cysts, cyst-like structures, and communicating and noncommunicating cysts is not possible because of the inability to differentiate true cysts from dilations of the subarachnoid space. MRI-based CSF-flow studies may be used in evaluation of cysts, in the postoperative period for follow-up after fenestration or marsupialization, and for differentiating normal dilation of CSF spaces from cysts.[40] This has only been evaluated in 1 case in the veterinary literature and the CSF flowed normally between the subarachnoid space and the SAD,

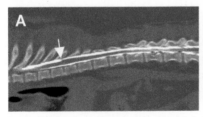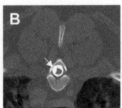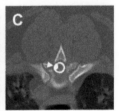

Fig. 7. (*A*) CT myelography of a French bulldog with an arachnoid diverticulum. (*A*) Sagittal CT myelographic image showing the tear-drop dilation of the subarachnoid space (*arrow*). (*B, C*) Transverse CT myelographic images showing the different appearances of the diverticulum (*arrows*).

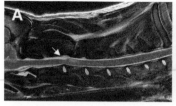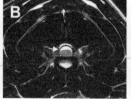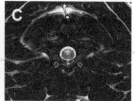

Fig. 8. Images of a 1 year-old American Pitbull with a cervical arachnoid diverticulum. (*A*) Sagittal T2-weighted image showing the diverticulum (*arrow*). (*B*) Transverse T2-weighted image at the C2-3 disc space showing the diverticulum (*arrow*). (*C*) Transverse T2-weighted image at the C3 region depicting the spinal cord hyperintensity suggestive of intramedullary edema.

leading the investigators to believe altered CSF flow was not responsible for formation of the SAD.[19]

CSF analysis is typically normal in most cases. Approximately 20% of dogs show albuminocytologic dissociation and 10% can show mild mononuclear pleocytosis.[1,18]

Histopathologic Findings

There is limited information about histopathology. In a case series by Gnirs and colleagues,[19] abnormal dural tissue was submitted for histopathology following durectomy. In 2 dogs, the dura and arachnoid layer were hypercellular with focal nodular aggregation. In 1 dog, the leptomeninges showed a cellular inflammatory reaction. In another dog, the leptomeninges revealed connective tissue proliferation with fibrosis and adhesion of the pia to the arachnoid layer. In 1 dog, the arachnoid membrane of the meningeal tissue was normal. In another case series, dural histopathology in 3 chondrodystrophic dogs with underlying intervertebral disc protrusions and SAD revealed primarily connective tissue proliferation with fibrosis.[41]

In 1 case series, 2 dogs were examined postmortem. In 1 dog that was euthanized for unrelated reasons 2 years postoperatively, the spinal cord at the site of the previously diagnosed SAD showed bilateral asymmetrical axonal degeneration and myelin loss with fibrous adhesion of the dorsal lamina to the dura mater. The second dog was euthanized 5 months postoperatively. Postmortem examination revealed marked dural and meningeal fibrosis with multifocal cystic cavitation of the dorsal funiculi.[18]

Treatment

Medical management (ie, glucocorticoid therapy) may be attempted initially. In a few cases, the signs can be managed for long periods and the disease seems to become

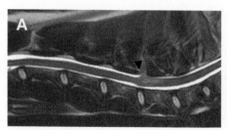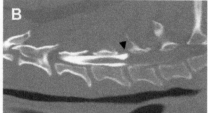

Fig. 9. Images of a Rottweiler dog with cervical arachnoid diverticulum. (*A*) Sagittal T2-weighted MRI. (*B*) CT myelogram image. Note that the diverticulum does not have the typical tear-drop appearance on MRI (*arrowheads*). CT myelography facilitates visualization and confirmation. (*From* Dewey CW, da Costa RC. Practical guide to canine and feline neurology. 3rd edition. Ames, IA: Wiley; 2016. p. 372; with permission.)

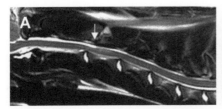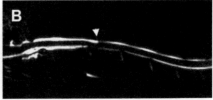

Fig. 10. MR images of a dog with an arachnoid diverticulum between C2 and C3. (*A*) Sagittal T2-weighted image (*arrow*) and (*B*) MR myelogram sequence (heavy T2, HASTE). Note that the diverticulum is more easily visualized in the MR myelogram sequence (*arrowhead*). (*From* Dewey CW, da Costa RC. Practical guide to canine and feline neurology. 3rd edition. Ames, IA: Wiley; 2016. p. 371; with permission.)

stable. Clinical signs in many dogs tend to be progressive and, therefore, surgical management is typically the treatment of choice. Surgical techniques described involved fenestration of the diverticulum with durotomy[19,24,41] or durectomy,[18,20,26–32,38,41,42] and marsupialization of the diverticulum.[20,21,43–45] In cases in which vertebral instability may be present, stabilization is recommended. Prognosis following surgery is difficult to interpret from the literature because of small case reports, varying treatment strategies, and limited follow-up. Surgical outcome is available from 3 case series.[18–20] The first study reported long-term outcome in 15 dogs treated surgically. Fourteen out of 15 dogs showed short-term improvement in clinical signs. Eight dogs (66%) were reported to have a successful long-term outcome with a median follow-up time of 23 months. Recurrence of signs was reported in 3 (25%) dogs but they occurred between 14 to 26 months following surgery.[20] Success rates were similar in the other 2 studies with 8 out of 12 (66%) and 7 out of 11 (64%).[18,19] From the limited data available, surgical treatment of spinal arachnoid cysts seems to have a good prognosis in many cases.[1,20] Ideal surgical technique is not known but 1 report suggests that marsupialization may have a slightly more favorable outcome than other techniques.[20] It is not clear how many dogs have recurrence because the follow-up of reported cases is variable; however, it seems that at least 10% to 20% of cases have recurrence of signs. Factors associated with a better outcome were age (younger than 3 years) and duration of clinical signs (less than 4 months).[20]

DISCAL CYSTS

Intraspinal cysts that arise from the disc have been uncommonly reported in dogs and humans.[46–49] There is some debate about whether these are truly discal cysts in dogs.[47,50] They are characterized by a capsule with serous or serosanguinous fluid that communicates with the intervertebral disc. They cause clinical signs similar to an acute disc extrusion, which is in contrast to presentation in humans in which there is usually chronic painful lumbar radiculopathy. Recently, the term acute compressive hydrated nucleus pulposus extrusion was suggested to describe dogs with these discal cyst type lesions.[51] Histopathology has not been done to confirm this hypothesis.[1] On MRI, they appear as cystic lesions dorsal to the intervertebral disc and cause deviation or deformation of the spinal cord. They are hyperintense in T2-weighted and hypointense on T1-weighted sequences, often with a contrast-enhancing rim. There may be a T2-weighted high intramedullary signal in the spinal cord suggestive of a contusion.[46,51] In a case series of 7 dogs, 6 cysts occurred in the cervical spine (C4-5 to C6-7) and 1 cyst was at T13-L1. Affected dogs were all more than 6 years of age with small and large breed dogs represented. All affected dogs were treated surgically. Rupture of the cyst with extravasation of its contents was achieved in all dogs with cervical discal cysts. The cyst was removed and evaluated histopathologically in only 1 dog with a T13-L1 cyst. The cyst wall was composed of irregular fibrous tissue consistent with fragments of annulus fibrosis and small parts of nucleus pulposus. Increased mucinous ground substance was observed within the annulus fibrosis. Nucleus pulposus was partially necrotic.[48] Recovery following surgery was satisfactory in all dogs.[47,48]

DERMOID SINUSES
Cause and Pathogenesis

A dermoid sinus is a blind tubular sac extending from dorsal midline ventrally into the underlying tissues. It is caused by incomplete separation of the neural tube from skin ectoderm during embryonic development.[17] It occurs most commonly in the cervical, thoracic, and lumbosacral spine.[52] This congenital anomaly was recognized as early as 1939 in South Africa, and later in the United States, in Rhodesian ridgeback dogs.[53,54] Other reported breeds include boerboel,[55] shih tzu,[56,57] chow chow,[58] Yorkshire terrier,[59] English springer spaniel,[60] golden retriever,[61] Great Pyrenees,[62] boxer,[57] and Siberian husky.[52] They are also reported in cats and Burmese cats seem to be predisposed.[63–69] It is inherited in Rhodesian ridgeback dogs as a dominant mutation in fibroblast growth factor genes.[70–72] The sinus tends to occur cranial or caudal to the ridge, particularly in the cervical or craniothoracic spine, but also occurs in the sacrococcygeal region or on the head. There are 4 types of dermoid sinuses described based on how deep into underlying tissues they extend (**Box 1, Fig. 11**).[52] Type V has been proposed but this represents a true cyst without a tract or opening.[17]

Clinical Signs

Clinical diagnosis is made by palpation of the dorsal midline defect and visual inspection by clipping the hair over the region of interest. The sinus tract often appears as a small (1–5 mm) indentation or invagination on the surface of the skin. On palpation it may feel like a cord or fibrous band passing subcutaneously. They can become inflamed and infected and will enlarge and become painful, sometimes with pyogranulomatous discharge.[17,52] Dogs with vertebral canal involvement may present with neurologic signs attributed to the location of the lesion, including ataxia, paresis, and/or hyperpathia. Myelitis or encephalitis may be present secondary to infection from the sinus.[52]

Diagnosis

In addition to physical examination findings, survey spinal radiographs may reveal dorsal lamina defects or osteomyelitis. Fistulography may be used to define the extent of the sinus. This is performed by infusing a sterile radiopaque water-soluble contrast

---

Box 1
Types of dermoid sinus

Type I: cylindrical sac extending to the supraspinous ligament

Type II: more superficial sac with a closed fibrous band extending to the supraspinous ligament

Type III: shallow superficial sac with no attachment to the supraspinous ligament

Type IV: extends to the vertebral canal with or without a lamina defect and often attaches to the dura mater

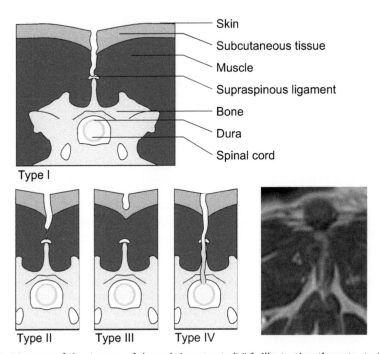

Type I

Type II   Type III   Type IV

Fig. 11. Diagram of the 4 types of dermal sinus tracts (I-IV), illustrating the extent of tissue depth involved. For comparison, a cervical transverse T2-weighted MRI of a type IV dermal sinus tract is shown. Note the serpentine appearance of the tract as it courses ventrally through a laminal defect to the dura mater. (*From* Westworth DR, Sturges BK. Congenital spinal malformations in small animals. Vet Clin North Am Small Anim Pract 2010;40(5):957; with permission; and [MRI] *Courtesy of* Dr Jim Lavely.)

medium via a catheter into the sinus opening. This may be helpful to determine the extent of the sinus before surgical excision.[52] There is some concern about introduction of infection into the CNS via fistulography and, therefore, it should be approached cautiously in cases with concern for spinal cord involvement.[17] MRI or CT is indicated when vertebral canal involvement is suspected. MRI may not always clearly indicate the full extent of the tract in certain cases.[73,74] If CNS infection is suspected, CSF should be obtained for cytologic evaluation and culture.[52]

Treatment

In some dogs, these sinuses do not cause clinical problems and do not require treatment. If they are infected, draining, or swollen, the treatment of choice is usually surgical excision. Cultures of tissues should be taken and antibiotic therapy prescribed if there is concern for infection.[17] Neurologic signs often improve after surgical removal of dermoid sinuses with vertebral canal involvement.[56,59,60,75,76] Histologically, these sinuses are lined with squamous epithelium, adnexal structures, epithelial debris, and inflammatory cells. *Staphylococcus intermedius* and *Enterococcus* spp are the most commonly isolated organisms.[17,52]

DERMOID AND EPIDERMOID CYSTS

Dermoid and epidermoid cysts are congenital inclusion cysts that arise from cutaneous ectodermal tissue trapped in the brain or spinal cord as a result of incomplete separation of neural ectoderm from cutaneous ectoderm at the time of neural tube closure. These are not the same as dermoid sinuses because they are restricted to the CNS and there is no tract or skin opening.[17] Both types of cysts are lined by keratinized, stratified squamous epithelium supported by a connective tissue stroma. Epidermoid cysts are similar to follicular dermal cysts and contain desquamated epithelial cells, keratin, and cholesterol. Dermal cysts also contain adnexal structures, such as sebaceous and apocrine glands, hair follicles, and fat.[77] These are rare congenital lesions in dogs.[78–81] MRI appearance was described in 1 case.[80] The cyst was hyperintense on T2-weighted images with hyperintensity of the spinal cord cranial to the cyst (consistent with edema) and ring enhancement on postcontrast T1-weighted images. Similar MRI features are described in humans and dogs with epidermoid cysts.[82–84] Reported cases in dogs have occurred in the thoracolumbar spine and clinical signs reflect the lesion location.[77,78] Treatment in humans is surgical removal with complete excision as a goal. At least 2 dogs in the literature had surgical removal with good outcomes.[77,81]

SUMMARY

Cystic lesions of the vertebral column and spinal cord are recognized with increasing frequency in domestic animals. Synovial cysts and arachnoid diverticula, in particular, are the most common of these cystic lesions. It is important that clinicians are aware of their location in the vertebral column, commonly affected breeds, and main clinical signs. The other cystic abnormalities described here (dermoid sinuses, dermoid and epidermoid cysts, and discal cysts) are encountered less commonly; however, with appropriate clinical suspicion, more of these diseases may be identified. The veterinary clinician should consider these diseases in the differential diagnoses of patients with signs of myelopathy.

REFERENCES

1. Lowrie ML, Platt SR, Garosi LS. Extramedullary spinal cysts in dogs. Vet Surg 2014;43(6):650–62.
2. Dickinson PJ, Sturges BK, Berry WL, et al. Extradural spinal synovial cysts in nine dogs. J Small Anim Pract 2001;42(10):502–9.
3. Hsu KY, Zucherman JF, Shea WJ, et al. Lumbar intraspinal synovial and ganglion cysts (facet cysts). Ten-year experience in evaluation and treatment. Spine (Phila Pa 1976) 1995;20(1):80–9.
4. Johnson JA, da Costa RC, Bhattacharya S, et al. Kinematic motion patterns of the cranial and caudal canine cervical spine. Vet Surg 2011;40(6):720–7.
5. Boviatsis EJ, Stavrinou LC, Kouyialis AT, et al. Spinal synovial cysts: pathogenesis, diagnosis and surgical treatment in a series of seven cases and literature review. Eur Spine J 2008;17(6):831–7.
6. Levitski RE, Chauvet AE, Lipsitz D. Cervical myelopathy associated with extradural synovial cysts in 4 dogs. J Vet Intern Med 1999;13(3):181–6.
7. Forterre F, Vizcaino Reves N, Stahl C, et al. Atlantoaxial synovial cyst associated with instability in a Chihuahua. Case Rep Vet Med 2012;2012:4.
8. Harris KP, Saveraid TC, Rodenas S. Dorsolateral spinal cord compression at the C2-C3 junction in two Cavalier King Charles spaniels. Vet Rec 2011;169(16):416.
9. Webb AA, Pharr JW, Lew LJ, et al. MR imaging findings in a dog with lumbar ganglion cysts. Vet Radiol Ultrasound 2001;42(1):9–13.
10. Forterre F, Kaiser S, Garner M, et al. Synovial cysts associated with cauda equina syndrome in two dogs. Vet Surg 2006;35(1):30–3.

11. Sale CS, Smith KC. Extradural spinal juxtafacet (synovial) cysts in three dogs. J Small Anim Pract 2007;48(2):116–9.
12. Perez B, Rollan E, Romiro, et al. Intraspinal synovial cyst in a dog. J Am Anim Hosp Assoc 2000;36(3):235–8.
13. Bley T, Lang J, Jaggy A, et al. Lumbar spinal 'juxtaarticular' cyst in a Gordon setter. J Vet Med A Physiol Pathol Clin Med 2007;54(9):494–8.
14. Lipsitz D, Levitski RE, Chauvet AE, et al. Magnetic resonance imaging features of cervical stenotic myelopathy in 21 dogs. Vet Radiol Ultrasound 2001;42(1): 20–7.
15. Martin-Vaquero P, da Costa RC. Magnetic resonance imaging features of Great Danes with and without clinical signs of cervical spondylomyelopathy. J Am Vet Med Assoc 2014;245(4):393–400.
16. Rohdin C, Nyman HT, Wohlsein P, et al. Cervical spinal intradural arachnoid cysts in related, young pugs. J Small Anim Pract 2014;55(4):229–34.
17. Westworth DR, Sturges BK. Congenital spinal malformations in small animals. Vet Clin North Am Small Anim Pract 2010;40(5):951–81.
18. Rylander H, Lipsitz D, Berry WL, et al. Retrospective analysis of spinal arachnoid cysts in 14 dogs. J Vet Intern Med 2002;16(6):690–6.
19. Gnirs K, Ruel Y, Blot S, et al. Spinal subarachnoid cysts in 13 dogs. Vet Radiol Ultrasound 2003;44(4):402–8.
20. Skeen TM, Olby NJ, Munana KR, et al. Spinal arachnoid cysts in 17 dogs. J Am Anim Hosp Assoc 2003;39(3):271–82.
21. Ness MG. Spinal arachnoid cysts in two shih tzu littermates. Vet Rec 1998; 142(19):515–6.
22. Nabors MW, Pait TG, Byrd EB, et al. Updated assessment and current classification of spinal meningeal cysts. J Neurosurg 1988;68(3):366–77.
23. Gage ED, Hoerlein BF, Bartels JE. Spinal cord compression resulting from a leptomeningeal cyst in the dog. J Am Vet Med Assoc 1968;152(11):1664–70.
24. Cambridge AJ, Bagley RS, Britt LG, et al. Radiographic diagnosis: arachnoid cyst in a dog. Vet Radiol Ultrasound 1997;38(6):434–6.
25. Mauler DA, De Decker S, De Risio L, et al. Signalment, clinical presentation, and diagnostic findings in 122 dogs with spinal arachnoid diverticula. J Vet Intern Med 2014;28(1):175–81.
26. Bagley RS, Silver GM, Seguin B, et al. Scoliosis and associated cystic spinal cord lesion in a dog. J Am Vet Med Assoc 1997;211(5):573–5.
27. Aikawa T, Kanazono S, Yoshigae Y, et al. Vertebral stabilization using positively threaded profile pins and polymethylmethacrylate, with or without laminectomy, for spinal canal stenosis and vertebral instability caused by congenital thoracic vertebral anomalies. Vet Surg 2007;36(5):432–41.
28. Galloway AM, Curtis NC, Sommerlad SF, et al. Correlative imaging findings in seven dogs and one cat with spinal arachnoid cysts. Vet Radiol Ultrasound 1999;40(5):445–52.
29. Schneider AR, Chen AV, Tucker RL. Imaging diagnosis–Vertebral canal porcupine quill with presumptive secondary arachnoid diverticulum. Vet Radiol Ultrasound 2010;51(2):152–4.
30. Chen AV, Bagley RS, West CL, et al. Fecal incontinence and spinal cord abnormalities in seven dogs. J Am Vet Med Assoc 2005;227(12):1945–51, 1928.
31. Jurina K, Grevel V. Spinal arachnoid pseudocysts in 10 rottweilers. J Small Anim Pract 2004;45(1):9–15.
32. Dyce J, Heritage ME, Houlton JEF, et al. Canine spinal 'arachnoid cysts'. J Small Anim Pract 1991;32(9):433–7.

33. Verhagen A, Go KG, Visser GM, et al. The presence of progesterone receptors in arachnoid granulations and in the lining of arachnoid cysts: its relevance to expression of progesterone receptors in meningiomas. Br J Neurosurg 1995; 9(1):47–50.
34. Go KG, Blankenstein MA, Vroom TM, et al. Progesterone receptors in arachnoid cysts. An immunocytochemical study in 2 cases. Acta Neurochir (Wien) 1997; 139(4):349–54.
35. Grant R, Condon B, Lawrence A, et al. Is cranial CSF volume under hormonal influence? An MR study. J Comput Assist Tomogr 1988;12(1):36–9.
36. Dewey CW, da Costa RC. Myelopathies: disorders of the spinal cord. In: Dewey CW, da Costa RC, editors. Practical guide to canine and feline neurology. 3rd edition. Ames, IA: Wiley; 2016.
37. Kendall BE, Valentine AR, Keis B. Spinal arachnoid cysts: clinical and radiological correlation with prognosis. Neuroradiology 1982;22(5):225–34.
38. Goncalves R, Hammond G, Penderis J. Imaging diagnosis: erroneous localization of spinal arachnoid cyst. Vet Radiol Ultrasound 2008;49(5):460–3.
39. Seiler GS, Robertson ID, Mai W, et al. Usefulness of a half-fourier acquisition single-shot turbo spin-echo pulse sequence in identifying arachnoid diverticula in dogs. Vet Radiol Ultrasound 2012;53(2):157–61.
40. Hoffmann KT, Hosten N, Meyer BU, et al. CSF flow studies of intracranial cysts and cyst-like lesions achieved using reversed fast imaging with steady-state precession MR sequences. AJNR Am J Neuroradiol 2000;21(3):493–502.
41. Frykman OF. Spinal arachnoid cyst in four dogs: diagnosis, surgical treatment and follow-up results. J Small Anim Pract 1999;40(11):544–9.
42. Sessums K, Mariani C. Intracranial meningioma in dogs and cats: a comparative review. Compend Contin Educ Vet 2009 Jul;31(7):330–9.
43. Oxley W, Pink J. Amelioration of caudal thoracic syringohydromyelia following surgical management of an adjacent arachnoid cyst. J Small Anim Pract 2012; 53(1):67–72.
44. McKee WM, Renwick PW. Marsupialisation of an arachnoid cyst in a dog. J Small Anim Pract 1994;35(2):108–11.
45. Bismuth C, Ferrand FX, Millet M, et al. Original surgical treatment of thoracolumbar subarachnoid cysts in six chondrodystrophic dogs. Acta Vet Scand 2014;56: 32.
46. Kono K, Nakamura H, Inoue Y, et al. Intraspinal extradural cysts communicating with adjacent herniated disks: imaging characteristics and possible pathogenesis. AJNR Am J Neuroradiol 1999;20(7):1373–7.
47. Penning VA, Benigni L, Steves E, et al. Imaging diagnosis–degenerative intraspinal cyst associated with an intervertebral disc. Vet Radiol Ultrasound 2007;48(5): 424–7.
48. Konar M, Lang J, Fluhmann G, et al. Ventral intraspinal cysts associated with the intervertebral disc: magnetic resonance imaging observations in seven dogs. Vet Surg 2008;37(1):94–101.
49. Kamishina H, Ogawa H, Katayama M, et al. Spontaneous regression of a cervical intraspinal cyst in a dog. J Vet Med Sci 2010;72(3):349–52.
50. Chiba K, Toyama Y, Matsumoto M, et al. Intraspinal cyst communicating with the intervertebral disc in the lumbar spine: discal cyst. Spine 2001;26(19): 2112–8.
51. Beltran E, Dennis R, Doyle V, et al. Clinical and magnetic resonance imaging features of canine compressive cervical myelopathy with suspected hydrated nucleus pulposus extrusion. J Small Anim Pract 2012;53(2):101–7.

52. Miller L, Tobias K. Dermoid sinuses: description, diagnosis, and treatment. Compend Contin Educ Vet 2003;25(4):295–300.
53. Steyn HP, Quinlan J, Jackson C. A skin condition seen in Rhodesian Ridgeback dogs: report on two cases. J S Afr Vet Assoc 1939;10(4):170–4.
54. Lord LH, Cawley AJ, Gilray J. Mid-dorsal dermoid sinuses in Rhodesian Ridgeback dogs; a case report. J Am Vet Med Assoc 1957;131(11):515–8.
55. Penrith ML, van Schouwenburg G. Dermoid sinus in a Boerboel bitch. J S Afr Vet Assoc 1994;65(2):38–9.
56. Colon JA, Maritato KC, Mauterer JV. Dermoid sinus and bone defects of the fifth thoracic vertebrae in a shih-tzu. J Small Anim Pract 2007;48(3):180.
57. Selcer EA, Helman RG, Selcer RR. Dermoid sinus in a shih tzu and a boxer. J Am Anim Hosp Assoc 1984;20:634–6.
58. Booth MJ. Atypical dermoid sinus in a chow chow dog. J S Afr Vet Assoc 1998; 69(3):102–4.
59. Fatone G, Brunetti A, Lamagna F, et al. Dermoid sinus and spinal malformations in a Yorkshire terrier: diagnosis and follow-up. J Small Anim Pract 1995;36(4): 178–80.
60. Pratt JN, Knottenbelt CM, Welsh EM. Dermoid sinus at the lumbosacral junction in an English springer spaniel. J Small Anim Pract 2000;41(1):24–6.
61. Cornegliani L, Jommi E, Vercelli A. Dermoid sinus in a golden retriever. J Small Anim Pract 2001;42(10):514–6.
62. Camacho AA, Laus JL, Veleri V. Dermoid sinus in a Great Pyrenees dog. Braz J Vet Res Anim Sci 1995;32:170–2.
63. Fleming JM, Platt SR, Kent M, et al. Cervical dermoid sinus in a cat: case presentation and review of the literature. J Feline Med Surg 2011;13(12):992–6.
64. Rochat MC, Campbell GA, Panciera RJ. Dermoid cysts in cats: two cases and a review of the literature. J Vet Diagn Invest 1996;8(4):505–7.
65. Henderson JP, Pearson GR, Smerdon TN. Dermoid cyst of the spinal cord associated with ataxia in a cat. J Small Anim Pract 1993;34(8):402–4.
66. Kiviranta AM, Lappalainen AK, Hagner K, et al. Dermoid sinus and spina bifida in three dogs and a cat. J Small Anim Pract 2011;52(6):319–24.
67. Tong T, Simpson DJ. Case report: Spinal dermoid sinus in a Burmese cat with paraparesis. Aust Vet J 2009;87(11):450–4.
68. Simpson D, Baral R, Lee D, et al. Dermoid sinus in Burmese cats. J Small Anim Pract 2011;52(11):616.
69. Akhtardanesh B, Kheirandish R, Azari O. Dermoid cyst in a domestic shorthair cat. Asian Pac J Trop Biomed 2012;2(3):247–9.
70. Salmon Hillbertz NH, Isaksson M, Karlsson EK, et al. Duplication of FGF3, FGF4, FGF19 and ORAOV1 causes hair ridge and predisposition to dermoid sinus in Ridgeback dogs. Nat Genet 2007;39(11):1318–20.
71. Salmon Hillbertz NH. Inheritance of dermoid sinus in the Rhodesian ridgeback. J Small Anim Pract 2005;46(2):71–4.
72. Salmon Hillbertz NH, Andersson G. Autosomal dominant mutation causing the dorsal ridge predisposes for dermoid sinus in Rhodesian ridgeback dogs. J Small Anim Pract 2006;47(4):184–8.
73. Rahal SC, Mortari AC, Yamashita S, et al. Magnetic resonance imaging in the diagnosis of type 1 dermoid sinus in two Rhodesian ridgeback dogs. Can Vet J 2008;49(9):871–6.
74. Davies ES, Fransson BA, Gavin PR. A confusing magnetic resonance imaging observation complicating surgery for a dermoid cyst in a Rhodesian Ridgeback. Vet Radiol Ultrasound 2004;45(4):307–9.

75. Ployart S, Doran I, Bomassi E, et al. Myelomeningocoele and a dermoid sinus-like lesion in a French bulldog. Can Vet J 2013;54(12):1133–6.
76. Barrios N, Gomez M, Mieres M, et al. Spinal dermoid sinus in a Dachshund with vertebral and thoracic limb malformations. BMC Vet Res 2014;10:54.
77. Cappello R, Lamb CR, Rest JR. Vertebral epidermoid cyst causing hemiparesis in a dog. Vet Rec 2006;158(25):865–7.
78. Hansmann F, Herder V, Ernst H, et al. Spinal epidermoid cyst in a SJL mouse: case report and literature review. J Comp Pathol 2011;145(4):373–7.
79. Lipitz L, Rylander H, Pinkerton ME. Intramedullary epidermoid cyst in the thoracic spine of a dog. J Am Anim Hosp Assoc 2011;47(6):e145–9.
80. Shamir MH, Lichovsky D, Aizenberg I, et al. Partial surgical removal of an intra-medullary epidermoid cyst from the spinal cord of a dog. J Small Anim Pract 1999;40(9):439–42.
81. Tshamala M, Moens Y. True dermoid cyst in a Rhodesian ridgeback. J Small Anim Pract 2000;41(8):352–3.
82. Bloomer CW, Ackerman A, Bhatia RG. Imaging for spine tumors and new applications. Top Magn Reson Imaging 2006;17(2):69–87.
83. Steinberg T, Matiasek K, Bruhschwein A, et al. Imaging diagnosis–intracranial epidermoid cyst in a Doberman Pinscher. Vet Radiol Ultrasound 2007;48(3):250–3.
84. Platt SR, Graham J, Chrisman CL, et al. Canine intracranial epidermoid cyst. Vet Radiol Ultrasound 1999;40(5):454–8.

Kyphosis and Kyphoscoliosis Associated with Congenital Malformations of the Thoracic Vertebral Bodies in Dogs

CrossMark

Curtis W. Dewey, DVM, MS[a],*, Emma Davies, BVSc, MSc[b],
Jennifer L. Bouma, VMD[c]

KEYWORDS

- Congenital • Malformation • Hemivertebrae • Thoracic • Kyphosis

KEY POINTS

- Malformations of the vertebral bodies often occur in the thoracic region of the vertebral column, primarily in small-breed dogs.
- These malformations are thought to represent errors in embryonic/fetal vertebral center ossification and/or fusion and typically result in kyphosis and scoliosis.
- The terms "hemivertebrae" and "butterfly" vertebrae are commonly, and often anatomically incorrectly, used to refer to these abnormalities; a more descriptive classification scheme has recently been reported.
- Most of these malformations are considered incidental findings, but some result in clinical signs of T3-L3 myelopathy of varying degrees of severity.

GENERAL OVERVIEW AND TERMINOLOGY

Malformations of the vertebral bodies in the thoracic spinal region of dogs are generally believed to be caused by failure of vertebral ossification centers to form, fuse properly, or both during embryonic or fetal development. The cause of this abnormal development is not fully understood, but such factors as genetic defects, teratogenic insults, and abnormal intersegmental blood supply to the developing vertebral column have been

The authors have nothing to disclose.

[a] Neurology/Neurosurgery Section, Department of Clinical Sciences, Cornell University Hospital for Animals, T6002C, Vet Research Tower, Ithaca, NY 14853, USA; [b] Neurology/Neurosurgery Section, Department of Clinical Sciences, Cornell University Hospital for Animals, College of Veterinary Medicine, Cornell University, T6002A, Vet Research Tower, Ithaca, NY 14853, USA; [c] Veterinary Specialists and Emergency Services, 825 White Spruce Boulevard, Suite 100, Rochester, NY 14623, USA
* Corresponding author.
E-mail address: cwd27@cornell.edu

implicated.[1–5] In humans with vertebral body malformations, genetic mutations have been identified in genes responsible for regulating normal fetal vertebral segmentation.[6] In humans and dogs, the vertebral malformations that tend to cause neurologic deficits are primarily those that lead to kyphosis (dorsal curvature) of the vertebral column.[3,5,7–9]

Terminology for the wide array of congenital vertebral anomalies encountered in small animal practice has been inconsistent and often confusing.[5] There are a variety of different shapes of aberrant vertebral bodies encountered in dogs with kyphosis, but the terms "hemivertebrae" and "butterfly vertebrae" are traditionally used to describe all of them.[1–3,8] Although incorrect, these two terms are sometimes used interchangeably in clinical parlance. A hemivertebra, or cuneiform vertebra, has been defined as one in which a portion of the vertebra fails to form correctly, resulting in a wedge shape to the vertebral body; the base of the wedge in most cases is oriented dorsally (**Fig. 1**).[1–3] This term, as it has been used most commonly, may also be an inaccurate description of most thoracic vertebral malformations that lead to neurologic dysfunction in dogs. A true hemivertebra is actually one where half of the vertebra (the centrum and neural arch) fails to form; this abnormality would lead to scoliosis, rather than kyphosis. The wedge-shaped thoracic "hemivertebra" typically encountered in clinically affected dogs is most likely caused by a failure of a portion of the body (centrum) of the vertebra to form, rather than representing a true hemivertebra.[5,10] When the central aspect of a vertebra fails to form, a more midline defect results, creating a shape that resembles the wings of a butterfly when viewed in a dorsal plane; this is the characteristic appearance of a "butterfly vertebra" (**Fig. 2**).[1,2,5,8,9] A more comprehensive radiographic classification system for thoracic vertebral anomalies in dogs has recently been proposed by Gutierrez-Quintana and colleagues,[8] and is based on schemes similar to those used in humans (**Fig. 3**). According to this scheme, kyphosis is more likely to develop with ventral hypoplasia (ventral wedge shape), ventral aplasia, and ventrolateral aplasia of the vertebral body. A butterfly vertebra is the result of ventral and median aplasia of the vertebra. In this study, dorsal and dorsolateral hemivertebrae (ventral and ventrolateral vertebral body aplasia, respectively) were more likely to be associated with neurologic deficits than other types of anomalies, including butterfly vertebrae.[8] The authors refer to abnormalities in this region of the vertebral column as congenital vertebral body malformations, and focus more on the individual shape of the abnormal region and effects on the spinal cord than specific terminology.

In both dogs and humans, the degree of kyphosis associated with the vertebral malformations determines the likelihood of developing neurologic dysfunction. Although some of these abnormalities often also produce some degree of scoliosis (lateral deviation of the vertebral column), this does not seem to have a substantial additional impact on the development of neurologic impairment.[5,7–9]

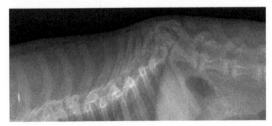

Fig. 1. Lateral radiograph of the vertebral column showing a hemivertebra or cuneiform vertebra at the level of T13. The malformation has resulted in a wedge-shaped vertebral body with the base oriented dorsally.

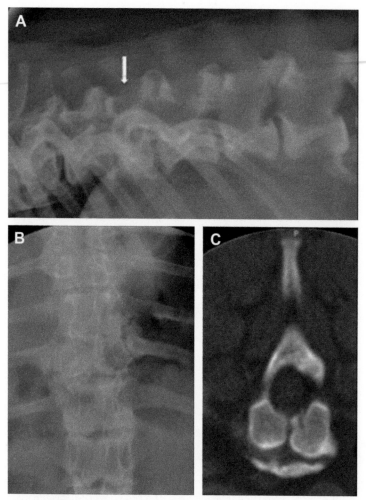

Fig. 2. Lateral (*A*) and dorsoventral (*B*) radiographs of the thoracic vertebral column showing a butterfly vertebra (*arrow* in *A*). (*C*) CT image showing the affected thoracic vertebra. The central vertebral body has failed to form resulting in the midline defect shown.

CLINICAL FEATURES

Thoracic vertebral body anomalies leading to kyphosis most commonly occur in small-breed dogs, particularly the brachycephalic "screw-tailed" breeds (English Bulldog, French Bulldog, Pug, Boston terrier). The abnormal shape of the tail in these breeds is thought to be caused by similar malformations in the coccygeal vertebral bodies.[1-5,7,8] These thoracic vertebral anomalies are occasionally encountered in other small-breed (eg, Yorkshire terrier, West Highland White terrier, Dachshund, Pekingese, Chihuahua, Maltese) and large-breed (eg, Doberman Pinscher, German Shorthaired Pointer) dogs. This is thought to be a heritable trait in the screw-tailed breeds and the disorder in German Shorthaired pointer dogs is believed to be auto-somal-recessive.[1-5,7,8] There is a wide age range at the time of clinical presentation, with about 60% being less than a year old and 40% greater than a year old.[11] There

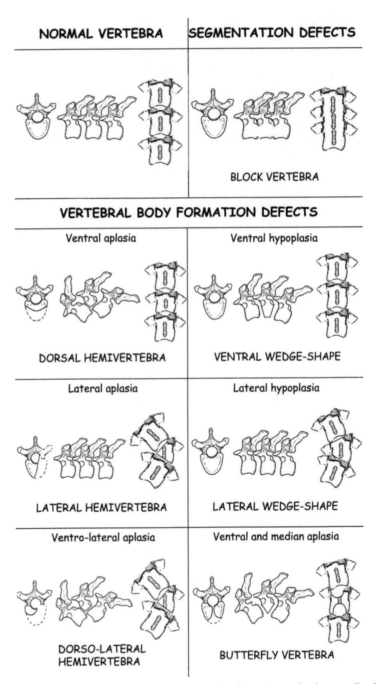

NORMAL VERTEBRA   **SEGMENTATION DEFECTS**

BLOCK VERTEBRA

VERTEBRAL BODY FORMATION DEFECTS

Ventral aplasia   Ventral hypoplasia

DORSAL HEMIVERTEBRA   VENTRAL WEDGE-SHAPE

Lateral aplasia   Lateral hypoplasia

LATERAL HEMIVERTEBRA   LATERAL WEDGE-SHAPE

Ventro-lateral aplasia   Ventral and median aplasia

DORSO-LATERAL
HEMIVERTEBRA   BUTTERFLY VERTEBRA

Fig. 3. Proposed radiographic classification system for thoracic vertebral anomalies in dogs based on schemes similar to those used in humans. (*From* Gutierrez-Quintana R, Guevar J, Stalin C, et al. A proposed radiographic classification scheme for thoracic vertebral malformations in brachycephalic "screw-tailed" dog breeds. Vet Radiol Ultrasound 2014;55(6):585–91; with permission.)

does not seem to be any obvious sex predilection for this disorder. In most cases, the malformed vertebra or vertebrae responsible for the deviation of the vertebral column are located in the mid to caudal thoracic vertebral region, usually between T6 and T9.[1,3,5,8,11] In one report,[8] the most commonly affected vertebra was T7, followed by T8 and T12.

Clinical signs of neurologic dysfunction are consistent with the location of the malformation, assuming that the thoracic vertebral malformation is the cause for the observed myelopathy. It is important for the clinician to remember that these malformations are often incidental findings and that there may be multiple malformations present in the same dog. It is also important to note that many of the breeds affected by thoracic vertebral malformations are also prone to other disorders of the thoracolumbar spine.[1] In particular, type I intervertebral disk extrusions are commonly encountered in most of the predisposed breeds. In one retrospective study comparing French Bulldogs and Dachshunds operated for type I disk extrusion, French Bulldogs with kyphotic thoracic vertebral anomalies were prone to disk extrusions in the L1-L5 vertebral segments; in these dogs, the abnormal thoracic vertebral segment was not considered of clinical significance.[12] If the thoracic vertebral malformation is the cause of neurologic dysfunction, the presentation is that of a T3-L3 myelopathy. Most dogs with clinical signs associated with a thoracic vertebral malformation present with a history of progressive ambulatory paraparesis and pelvic limb ataxia, which may wax and wane. Occasionally, a dog with a thoracic vertebral malformation presents as an acute-onset T3-L3 myelopathy, and some may be nonambulatory paraparetic or paraplegic. Also, some dogs with chronic, progressive signs of ambulatory paraparesis may acutely decompensate and become nonambulatory.[1–3,5,8,11,12] There may be evidence of hyperesthesia in the region of the spinal deformity, and some owners state they believe their pet is experiencing back pain. The kyphotic vertebral segment in affected dogs is believed to result in compression of the spinal cord in that region; also, it is suspected that the area in the vicinity of the abnormal vertebrae is a site of instability, which can result in repeated trauma to the spinal cord in the region of the vertebral deformity.[1–3,8,11–13]

DIAGNOSTIC IMAGING

The imaging modalities available (**Box 1**) for diagnosing and characterizing congenital thoracic vertebral body abnormalities in dogs include radiography, myelography, computed tomography (CT), and MRI.[1,5,13–15] The presence of vertebral anomalies and the degree of associated kyphosis (lateral view) and scoliosis (dorsoventral view) are readily appreciated on survey radiographs of the spine (**Fig. 4**). As previously mentioned, scoliosis is typically not associated with neurologic dysfunction. The degree of kyphosis has been associated with the presence of neurologic dysfunction

Box 1
Imaging modalities
Radiography
Myelography
CT
MRI
Multiple modalities

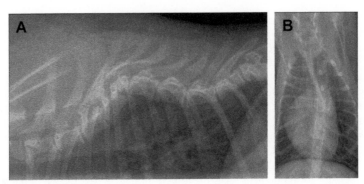

Fig. 4. Thoracic vertebral malformation resulting in (*A*) kyphosis shown on the lateral radiograph and (*B*) scoliosis shown on the dorsoventral radiograph of the thoracic vertebral column.

in dogs and humans.[3,7–9] The degree of angulation of the vertebral segment associated with the anomalous vertebra or vertebrae is quantified by measuring the Cobb angle. The Cobb angle is derived from the intersection of two lines: one at the cranial aspect of the kyphotic vertebral segment and the other at the caudal aspect of the segment (**Fig. 5**).[7,12] In one retrospective study, a significant difference in kyphotic Cobb angles was appreciated between dogs with and without neurologic dysfunction; most dogs with neurologic dysfunction had a Cobb angle associated with the kyphotic vertebral segment greater than 35°.[7]

Radiographs provide evidence of bony malformation, but do not provide information regarding the presence and degree of spinal cord compression or the presence of other possible parenchymal lesions in the spinal cord (eg, syringomyelia, arachnoid diverticula). Myelography can provide evidence of spinal cord compression, but some parenchymal spinal cord abnormalities, if present, may not be visible on myelography. MRI provides superior parenchymal detail, and is the best imaging choice to investigate for evidence of spinal cord compression and the presence of potential accompanying spinal cord abnormalities (**Fig. 6**). T1-weighted sequences

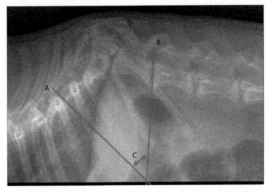

Fig. 5. Lateral thoracic radiograph from a dog with a vertebral malformation showing the Cobb angle of 47° (C) at the intersection of two lines (A) cranial and (B) caudal to the malformation.

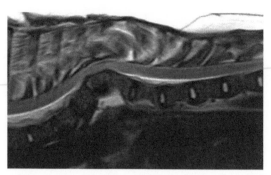

Fig. 6. Sagittal T2-weighted MRI of the thoracic spine showing a T5 vertebral malformation with the kyphosis resulting in compression of the spinal cord.

are preferable for bone detail in MRIs. Bony detail and the three-dimensional (3D) trajectory of the vertebral column in all planes is best achieved via CT, including 3D reconstructed CT images (**Fig. 7**).[1,5,15] In cases of thoracic vertebral anomalies for which surgery is likely, the authors prefer MRI, followed by CT imaging of the specific segment of interest. Creating a 3D plastic model of an individual patient's specific vertebral region of interest (**Fig. 8**) can be invaluable in presurgical planning, especially if vertebral body implants are going to be placed.

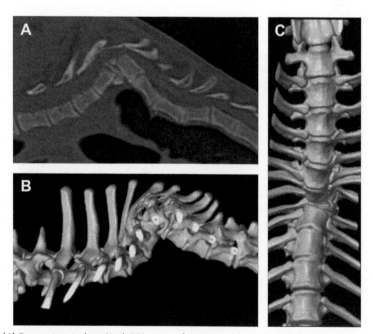

Fig. 7. (*A*) Reconstructed sagittal CT image of a young dog with a thoracic vertebral malformation. Lateral (*B*) and ventral (*C*) views of 3D reconstructed CT images in the same dog, which allows better visualization of bone trajectories.

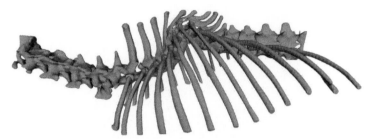

Fig. 8. A 3D sagittal computer-aided design model from CT images of a young dog with a thoracic vertebral malformation. The model can then be used to print a 3D solid object to aid in visualization and surgical planning.

MEDICAL MANAGEMENT

Medical management is instituted in clinically affected dogs, whether or not surgical correction of the deformity is planned. Medical management typically consists of anti-inflammatory doses of prednisone, strict exercise restriction (with potential crate confinement), and pain-relieving drugs (**Box 2**). Nonsteroidal anti-inflammatory drugs are appropriate for dogs experiencing clinical signs of back pain with minimal to no pelvic limb motor deficits. In the authors' experience, prednisone is more effective than nonsteroidal anti-inflammatory drugs in managing dogs with obvious motor dysfunction, presumably via its ability to reduce edema. In young ambulatory patients with nonprogressive signs of myelopathy, it may be worth postponing surgery until after 9 months of age (the approximate age at which vertebral growth ceases). In some of these younger patients, clinical signs may eventually stabilize or even improve.[11,14] In the face of progressive and severe myelopathy that causes obvious dysfunction, surgical correction should be considered irrespective of age.[11,13–15] In those cases for which surgery is not a viable option because of financial limitations or other health-related issues, prolonged medical management may be necessary to try to preserve adequate function and patient comfort for as long as possible.

SURGICAL MANAGEMENT

The goals of surgical management are to relieve spinal cord compression in the region of the kyphotic vertebral segment and stabilize the abnormal vertebral region.[1,11,13–15] There are few published reports detailing surgical management of

Box 2
Medical management

Medical Management	Doses
Nonsteroidal anti-inflammatory drugs (eg, carprofen)	4 mg/kg/d PO divided Q12–24 h for 7 d 2 mg/kg/d PO Q24 h for another 7 d
Prednisone (anti-inflammatory)	0.5 mg/kg PO Q12–24 h, taper
Gabapentin	10–60 mg/kg/d PO divided Q8–12 h (start at 10 mg/kg Q8 h and titrate up to effect)
Pregabalin	2–4 mg/kg PO Q8 h (start at 2 mg/kg and titrate up to effect)
Amantadine	3–5 mg/kg PO Q24 h

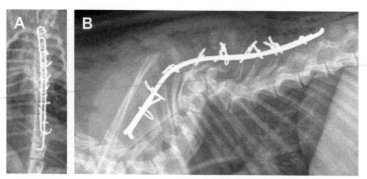

Fig. 9. Ventrodorsal (*A*) and lateral (*B*) radiographs showing postoperative segmental spinal implants to stabilize the vertebral column in a young dog with a thoracic vertebral malformation. Images show the use of wire to stabilize the segments. (*Courtesy* of N. Jeffrey, BVSc, PhD, DECVS, DECVN, SAS, FRCVS, Iowa State University College of Veterinary Medicine, Ames, IA.)

this disorder; therefore, surgical recommendations of the authors are based on a combination of the existing literature and personal experience.[11,13–15] The authors consider the abnormal vertebral segment to be unstable in dogs with clinical dysfunction associated with vertebral body malformations. We also believe that decompression is usually indicated over the region of spinal cord impingement, either via a dorsal laminectomy or hemilaminectomy. The two main methods of stabilizing kyphotic vertebral segments in these patients is via segmental spinal stabilization (often referred to as spinal "stapling"; **Fig. 9**), and vertebral body pin and polymethylmethacrylate fixation (**Fig. 10**).[11,13–15] Successful outcomes have been reported in most dogs treated with either of these methods.[11,13–15] A major challenge in placing vertebral body pins in dogs with deformed vertebrae is accounting for the various planes in which the vertebral column traverses when placing pins in the vertebral body. A very narrow passageway exists for optimal placement of these pins (**Fig. 11**); an error in either direction may result in either inadequate bone purchase or entry into the vertebral canal. In humans with severe kyphotic vertebral malformations in the thoracic region, achieving sagittal realignment with surgery is

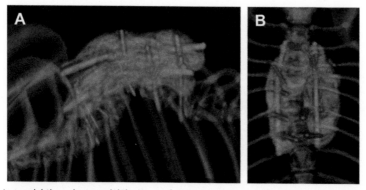

Fig. 10. Lateral (*A*) and ventral (*B*) views of 3D reconstructed CT images showing postoperative vertebral body pin and polymethylmethacrylate stabilization following dorsal laminectomy to decompress the spinal cord in a young dog with a thoracic vertebral malformation.

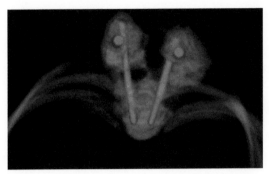

Fig. 11. Transverse view of 3D reconstructed CT image showing postoperative vertebral body pin and polymethylmethacrylate stabilization following dorsal laminectomy.

typically a major objective, considering the upright posture of this species. To achieve this goal, procedures that entail removal of sections of vertebral bodies (osteomies) or entire vertebral bodies (corpectomies) to realign the vertebral column are often entailed.[16] In the authors' opinion, such realignment procedures are generally unnecessary in dogs with kyphotic malformations, considering this species' quadrupedal stance.

The authors prefer a surgical technique that is a hybrid of the two techniques most commonly used for this condition (**Fig. 12**). A hemilaminectomy is performed over the kyphotic segment. Vertebral body pins are placed in the side of the hemilaminectomy and a spinal staple is placed on the opposite side. In this method, the trajectory of the spinal cord is visualized while placing vertebral body pins. Regardless of the surgical method of vertebral stabilization chosen, either postoperative radiographs or CT imaging is recommended to assess the adequacy of implant placement.

Postsurgically, patients need to be confined to a crate, with short leash walks only (to urinate and defecate) for 4 to 6 weeks. After this time period, a gradual return to normal activity is encouraged. Anti-inflammatory and analgesic therapy is gradually withdrawn 1 to 2 weeks postoperatively.

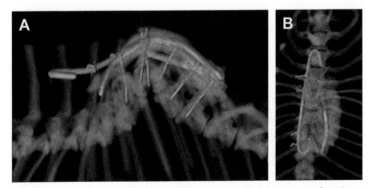

Fig. 12. Lateral (*A*) and ventral (*B*) views of 3D reconstructed CT images showing postoperative hybrid stabilization using two of the most common techniques following hemilaminectomy to decompress the spinal cord in a young dog with a thoracic vertebral malformation.

SUMMARY

Malformations of the vertebral bodies often occur in the thoracic region of the vertebral column, primarily in small-breed dogs. These malformations are thought to represent errors in embryonic/fetal vertebral center ossification and/or fusion and typically result in kyphosis and scoliosis. The terms "hemivertebrae" and "butterfly" vertebrae are commonly, and often anatomically incorrectly, used to refer to these abnormalities; a more descriptive classification scheme has recently been reported. Most of these malformations are considered incidental findings, but some result in clinical signs of T3-L3 myelopathy of varying degrees of severity. Some dogs are managed medically, whereas others require surgery to prevent permanent pelvic limb dysfunction. A combination of MRI and CT imaging is beneficial to diagnosis and surgical planning. Several methods of surgical correction have been described, all of which seem to result in a favorable outcome in most cases.

REFERENCES

1. Dewey CW, da Costa RC. Myelopathies: disorders of the spinal cord. In: Dewey CW, da Costa RC, editors. Practical guide to canine and feline neurology. 3rd edition. Ames (IA): Wiley-Blackwell; 2016. p. 329–403.
2. Bailey CS, Morgan JP. Congenital spinal malformations. Vet Clin Small Anim 1992;22:985–1015.
3. Moissonnier P, Gossot P, Scotti S. Thoracic kyphosis associated with hemivertebra. Vet Surg 2011;40:1029–32.
4. Besalti O, Ozak A, Pekcan Z, et al. Nasca classification of hemivertebra in five dogs. Ir Vet J 2005;58:688–90.
5. Westworth DR, Sturges BK. Congenital spinal malformations in small animals. Vet Clin Small Anim 2010;40:951–81.
6. Pourquié O, Kusumi K. When body segmentation goes wrong. Clin Genet 2001; 60:409–16.
7. Guevar J, Penderis J, Faller K, et al. Computer-assisted radiographic calculation of spinal curvature in brachycephalic "screw-tailed" dog breeds with congenital thoracic vertebral malformations: reliability and clinical evaluation. PLoS One 2014;9(9):e106957.
8. Gutierrez-Quintana R, Guevar J, Stalin C, et al. A proposed radiographic classification scheme for congenital thoracic vertebral malformations in brachycephalic "screw-tailed" dog breeds. Vet Radiol Ultrasound 2014;55: 585–91.
9. McMaster MJ, Singh H. Natural history of congenital kyphosis and congenital scoliosis. J Bone Joint Surg Am 1999;81(10):1367–83.
10. Hedequist D, Emans J. Congenital scoliosis: a review and update. J Pediatr Orthop 2007;27:106–16.
11. Charalambous M, Jeffery ND, Smith PM, et al. Surgical treatment of dorsal hemivertebrae associated with kyphosis by spinal segmental stabilization, with or without decompression. Vet J 2014;202:267–73.
12. Aikawa T, Shibata M, Asano M, et al. A comparison of thoracolumbar intervertebral disc extrusion in French Bulldogs and Dachshunds and association with congenital vertebral anomalies. Vet Surg 2014;43:301–7.
13. Aikawa T, Kanazono S, Yoshigae Y, et al. Vertebral stabilization using positively threaded profile pins and polymethylmethacrylate, with or without laminectomy, for spinal canal stenosis and vertebral instability caused by congenital thoracic vertebral anomalies. Vet Surg 2007;36:432–41.

14. Jeffery ND, Smith PM, Talbot CE. Imaging findings and surgical treatment of hemivertebrae in three dogs. J Am Vet Med Assoc 2007;230:532–6.

15. Dewey CW. Surgery of the thoracolumbar spine. In: Fossum TW, editor. Small animal surgery. St Louis (MO): Elsevier; 2013. p. 1508–28.

16. Yaman O, Dalbayrak S. Kyphosis and review of the literature. Turk Neurosurg 2014;24:455–65.

Congenital Malformations of Vertebral Articular Processes in Dogs

 CrossMark

Jennifer L. Bouma, VMD

KEYWORDS

- Congenital • Malformation • Articular process • Articular facet
- Articular process dysplasia • Caudal articular process aplasia
- Caudal articular process hypoplasia • Pug

KEY POINTS

- Congenital anomalies of the articular processes in dogs are not necessarily incidental.
- The introduction and widespread use of advanced cross-sectional imaging such as computed tomography and MRI in academic as well as private veterinary practice have allowed for detailed evaluation of the spine, spinal cord, and nerve roots.
- The clinical relevance and clinical manifestation of articular processes anomalies are heavily dependent on location within the spine.
- Although no definitive cause has been identified, the breed-specific anomalies of articular processes that have thus far been identified are strong indicators of a genetic component.

ANATOMY AND PHYSIOLOGY REVIEW

The spine is divided into 5 regions: cervical, thoracic, lumbar, sacrum, and caudal/coccygeal. The standard formula for the spine of the domestic dog is C7, T13, L7, and S3. There are a variable number of caudal vertebra. All vertebral bodies have the same basic components: body, arch, and paired articular processes (**Fig. 1**). The arch is composed of paired pedicles and laminae. Articular processes are located at the cranial and caudal surfaces of the vertebra and arise from the junction of the pedicle and lamina[1] (**Fig. 2**).

The vertebral canal is formed by fusion of the vertebral body and arch; the canal protects the spinal cord and spinal nerve roots. As a whole, the vertebral column supports the head and provides attachment of major muscle groups. With the exception of the fused sacrum, all vertebrae are separate from one another and articulate with adjacent

The author has nothing to disclose.
Veterinary Specialists & Emergency Services, 825 White Spruce Boulevard, Suite 100, Rochester, NY 14623, USA
E-mail address: jenniferbouma@yahoo.com

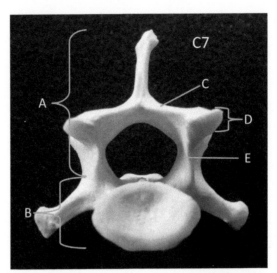

Fig. 1. Caudal view of the seventh cervical vertebra. All vertebral bodies have the same basic components: (A) arch, (B) body, (C) lamina, (D) paired articular processes, (E) pedicle. (Please note that only the caudal articular processes are labeled in this image [D]. The cranial articular processes are not visible due to superimposition.)

vertebral bodies via synovial joints to form movable joints.[1,2] In conjunction with soft tissue structures of the spine, the articular process joint functions to provide stable flexibility between the vertebral bodies.[1–5] The articular processes contribute up to 30% of the stability of the vertebral column.[6,7] The articular processes in the cranial thoracic spine (T1-T9) also function in weight-bearing.[3]

Motion of the spine is governed by orientation of the corresponding caudal and cranial articular processes. Although as a whole, the vertebral column of the dog is flexible, the range of motion for individual articular process joints is limited by comparison.[1,2] The basic movements of the vertebral column include dorsal arching; extension; ventral arching; lateral flexion; and rotation.[1] With the exception of C1 and C2, the cranial and caudal articular processes of the entire vertebral column have orientation that may be classified into 1 of 2 categories. Cranial processes will be either craniodorsal or medial; caudal processes are caudoventral or lateral[1] (**Fig. 3**).

In locations of the vertebral column where stability is imperative, mobility of the adjacent vertebral bodies is limited by opposing incline of articulating caudal and cranial processes. Examples include the atlanto-axial articulation, cervical-thoracic (CT) junction, and the anticlinal space[1] (**Fig. 4**). The most flexible locations of the spine have the most voluminous articular capsules to allow for the greatest range of motion. These locations include the base of the tail and the cervical region (**Fig. 5A**).[2]

The Cervical Vertebrae

There is little variation of the anatomy of the articular processes of C3-C7. The caudal articular processes have caudoventral orientation, and cranial articular processes are oriented in corresponding craniodorsal direction[1] (see **Figs. 2** and **3**). Cervical articular process joint capsules are voluminous, allowing for large range of motion.[2]

In addition to the readily identifiable unique shapes of C1 and C2, their articulation is also different. Congenital anomalies of the atlanto-axial and atlanto-occipital articulations are covered in a separate article.

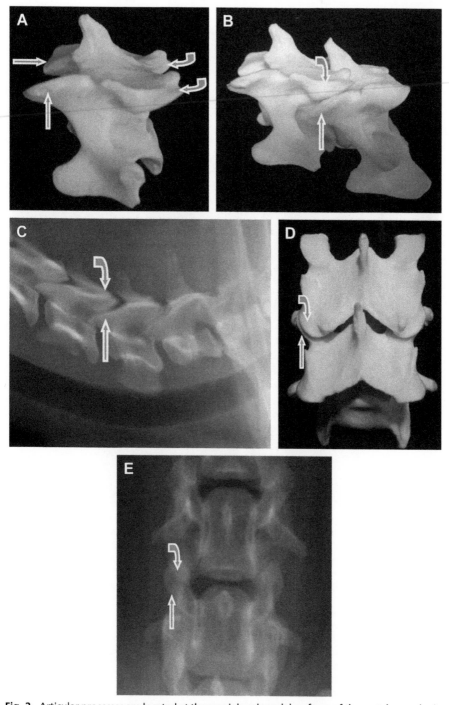

Fig. 2. Articular processes are located at the cranial and caudal surfaces of the vertebra and arise from the junction of pedicle and lamina. The articular surfaces of the cranial articular processes of C3-C7 are craniodorsal. The articular surface of the caudal articular processes of C3-C7 are caudoventral. Cranial articular processes in these images are labeled with straight arrows, and caudal articular processes are labeled with curved arrows. (*A*) Lateral view of C5 bone specimen; (*B*) lateral view of bone specimen, C5-C6 articulation; (*C*) lateral radiograph C4-T1; (*D*) dorsal view of bone specimen, C5-C6 articular process joints; (*E*) ventrodorsal radiograph of C5-C6 articulation.

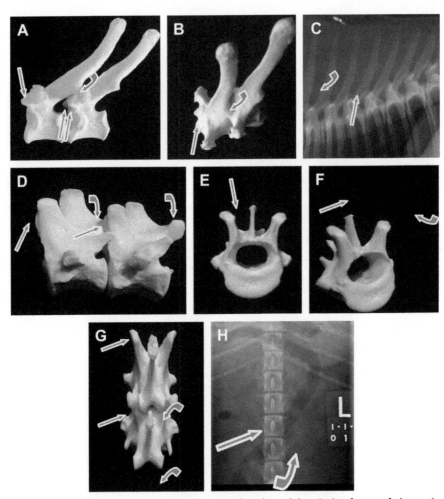

Fig. 3. With the exception of C1-C2, the cranial and caudal articular facets of the entire spine will have orientation that falls into 1 of 2 categories. Cranial articular facets will be either craniodorsal or medial; caudal processes will be caudoventral or lateral. Cranial articular facets in these images are labeled with straight arrows, and caudal articular facets are labeled with curved arrows. For T1-T9, the articular surfaces of the cranial articular facets are dorsal; articular surfaces of the caudal facets are ventral. For T10, articular surfaces of the cranial facets are dorsal and articular surfaces of the caudal facets are lateral. For T11-T13, the articular surfaces of the cranial facets are medial and articular surfaces of the caudal facets are lateral. (A) Lateral view of T6-T7 bone specimen; (B) dorsolateral oblique view of T6-T7 bone specimen; (C) lateral radiograph of T6-T7; (D) lateral view of T12-T13 bone specimen; (E) cranial view of T12 bone specimen; (F) craniolateral oblique projection of T12 bone specimen highlighting the medial articular surface of the cranial articular facet; (G) dorsal view of T12-T13 bone specimen, the lateral articular surface of T12 caudal articular facet articulates with medial articular surface of cranial articular facet T13; (H) ventrodorsal radiograph of caudal aspect of T11–mid L2.

The size and shape of the vertebral canal reflect the size and shape of the cord at that location.[1,8] The canal has a round shape within C1-C3. The canal enlarges and changes into an ovoid shape from C4 into the cranial thoracic spine, T2, to accommodate the cervical intumescence.[1,8] The canal is the largest overall within the atlas,

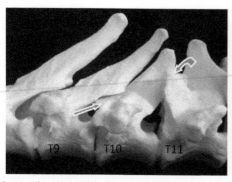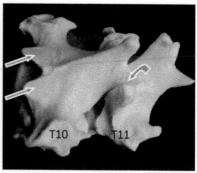

Fig. 4. The anticlinal space, T10-T11 is an example of a portion of the spine with opposing incline of cranial and caudal articular processes that provides stability. T10 represents a transition in the orientation of the articular processes of the thoracic spine. The articular surface of the cranial process of T10 is dorsal and the articular surface of the caudal process is lateral. In these images of bone specimens, the cranial articular process is identified with straight arrows, and the caudal articular process is identified with curved arrows.

which corresponds to largest (height) diameter of the cord.[1] The cord tapers to half of its height within the caudal aspect of the axis. Despite large breed differences in the overall size of the canine skeleton, the circumference of the cord[1] does not vary (if at all), but the dimensions of the canal are more proportional to patient size. This difference can be significant in certain disease processes in which the dimensions of the canal are compromised. What might be a minor extradural compressive lesion in a large or giant breed dog is translated into a major source of compression for a small breed dog.

Thoracic Vertebrae

Although the anatomy of the first nine thoracic vertebrae is similar, the wide separation of the cranial articular processes of T1 and T2 is a dramatic contrast from T3-T9, which are almost confluent in the median plane (**Figs. 5**B and **6**). The orientation of the articular

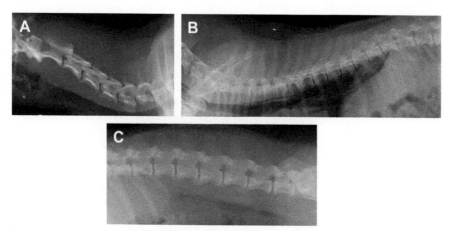

Fig. 5. (*A*) Lateral radiograph of the normal canine cervical spine. (*B*) Lateral radiograph of the normal canine thoracic spine. (*C*) Lateral radiograph of the normal lumbar spine.

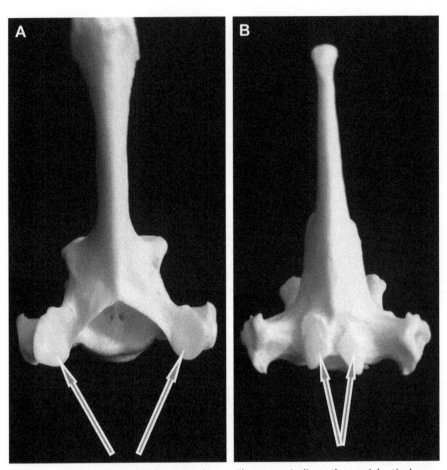

Fig. 6. Dorsal view of T1 and T7 bone specimens. The arrows indicate the cranial articular processes, which face dorsally in both vertebra. (*A*) Notice how separated the left and right articular processes of T1 are positioned. (*B*) In contrast, the dorsal articular processes of T7 are very close to one another, almost confluent.

surfaces of cranial articular processes of T1-T9 is craniodorsal. The articular surfaces of the caudal articular processes of T1-T9 have a similar shape compared with the cranial processes, but their orientation is in a corresponding caudoventral direction. This "tiled" orientation of the articular processes of the cranial two-thirds of the thoracic spine helps function in weight-bearing, which is unique in this portion of the vertebral column[3] (**Fig. 7**).

The final 4 thoracic vertebra represent a transitional portion of the spine. The orientations of the articular surfaces of the cranial and caudal articular processes of T10-T13 are summarized in **Table 1**. In contrast to the tiled arrangement of the prediaphragmatic thoracic vertebrae, the caudal thoracic articular process joints are modified. The articular surfaces cranial articular processes of T10 are dorsal and nearly confluent on the median plane, similar to the prediaphragmatic portion of the thoracic spine. The caudal articular process of T10 is on the sagittal plane and the articular surface faces laterally. The caudal articular processes of T11-lumbar spine are similar to T10, but the

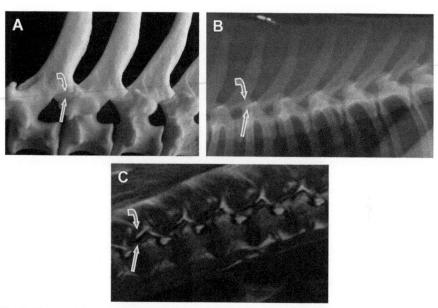

Fig. 7. The cranial and caudal articular processes of T1-T9 have similar shape. Articular surfaces of the cranial processes are craniodorsal, and articular surfaces of the caudal processes have corresponding caudoventral orientation. This tiled arrangement help in weight-bearing. Cranial articular processes in these images are labeled with straight arrows, and caudal articular processes are labeled with curved arrows. (*A*) Lateral view of cranial thoracic spine, bone specimen. (*B*) Lateral radiographic projection of the cranial thoracic spine. (*C*) T1-weighted sagittal sequence of the cranial thoracic spine.

Table 1
Orientation of dorsal spinous processes, articular surface of the cranial articular processes, and articular surface of the caudal articular processes of the postdiaphragmatic thoracic spine (T10-T13)

	Cranial Articular Processes	Caudal Articular Processes	Dorsal Spinous Processes

T10
Diaphragmatic vertebra
	Dorsal
	Nearly confluent on
	    median plane
		Lateral	Slight caudal
			    orientation

T11
Anticlinal vertebra
	Dorsal
	Adjacent to the
	    mammillary processes
	Face one another across
	    midline
		Lateral	Perpendicular
			    orientation

T12	Dorsal
	Adjacent to the
	    mammillary processes
	Face one another across
	    midline
		Lateral	Cranial orientation

T13	Dorsal
	Adjacent to the
	    mammillary processes
	Face one another across
	    midline
		Lateral	Cranial orientation

articular surface of the cranial articular processes are also dorsal (see **Fig. 3**). The caudal articular surfaces of T10-T13 are medial, facing one another across midline to form an interlocking network in the sagittal plane, which restricts lateral flexion.

The orientation of the dorsal spinous processes from T1-T7 are in the caudal direction. As the orientation of the articular process joints shifts, there is a corresponding change in the angulation of the dorsal spinous processes. There is a gradual shift in the orientation of the dorsal spinous processes of T8 and T9. The most notable change is located, as the name suggests, at the anticlinal space: T10-T11. The diaphragmatic vertebra,[9] T10, is the last thoracic vertebral body that has a dorsal spinous process with caudal orientation. The dorsal spinous process of T11, the anticlinal vertebra, has perpendicular orientation. The dorsal spinous processes of T12 and T13 have a slight cranial orientation (see **Fig. 5B**).

Accessory processes are present from the midthoracic spine and may continue as far caudal as L5 or L6. Accessory processes arise from the caudal lateral border of the pedicle and are oriented in a caudal and dorsal direction. When well-developed, the cranial base of the cranial articular process of the adjoining vertebra will fit into the lateral ventral notch created by the space between the pedicle and the accessory process[1] (**Fig. 8**). The presence of a well-developed accessory process can aid in the stabilization of the spine and restrict lateral bending. The variable presence or absence of accessory processes may help explain differences in clinical relevance of articular process dysplasia, but this is an area that will require further review.

The vertebral canal within T1 and T2 is large and ovoid to accommodate the caudal portion of the cervical intumescence as previously mentioned. The canal changes to circular shape and is uniform in size from T3-T11.[1] From T11-L6, there is no change in height, but there is an increase in width of the canal. Thus, the shape of the canal changes yet again from round to ovoid shape.

Lumbar Vertebrae

The articular processes of the entire lumbar vertebral column are uniform. Similar to the caudal thoracic spine, the articular process joints form an interlocking sagittal plane, which restricts lateral flexion (see **Fig. 4**; **Fig. 5C**). The articular surfaces of the cranial articular processes are dorsal-medial, and the articular surfaces of the caudal articular processes are dorsal-lateral. The accessory processes of L1-L3 and occasionally L4 are well developed. Accessory processes are often absent on L5 and L6.

The canal remains ovoid in shape from caudal thorax into the lumbar spine. The diameter is largest within bodies of L6-L7 to accommodate the lumbar intumescence.

ARTICULAR PROCESS DYSPLASIA

Most articular process anomalies have been considered congenital in nature.[3–5,10–14] However, like many congenital spinal anomalies, the recurrence of congenital anomalies in specific breeds may be indicative of genetic predispositions that are yet to be determined.[3–5,10–24] The clinical significance of these anomalies varies and is interdependent on 3 factors: location (cervical, thoracic, and lumbosacral), function (mobility, stabilization, and weight-bearing), and anatomy (variations of articular process conformation and variations in shape and size of the vertebral canal).

The proposed definition of articular process dysplasia comprises a spectrum of congenital anomalies affecting either cranial or caudal articular process. These anomalies include absent process (aplasia); incomplete (hypoplasia) process formation; and enlarged (hyperplastic) process formation (**Figs. 9** and **10**). With the aid of advanced cross-sectional imaging (MRI and CT), constrictive myelopathy, a clinically relevant

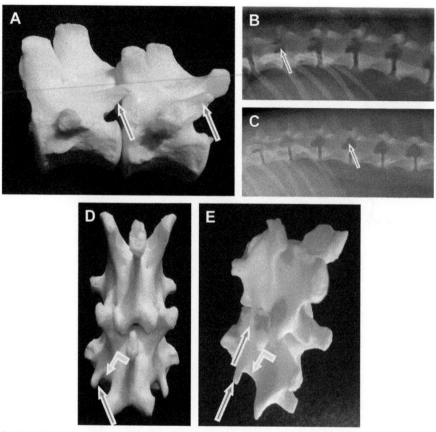

Fig. 8. When present, the paired accessory processes arise from the caudal lateral border of the pedicle in the midthoracic spine and continue as far caudal as L5-L6. They are oriented in the caudodorsal direction. The base of the cranial articular process of the adjoining vertebra fits into the "U-shaped" notch created between the pedicle and the accessory process. In dogs with well-developed accessory processes, this notch provides additional stabilization in lateral movement of the spine. In these images, the accessory process is identified with the straight arrow, and the notch is identified with the bent arrow. (*A*) Lateral aspect of bone specimen T12-T13. Arrows identify well-developed accessory processes on both T12 and T13. (*B*) Lateral radiograph of the thoracolumbar (TL) spine in a dog with well-developed accessory processes. It is interesting to note that the T12 caudal articular process is aplastic and T13 is hypoplastic. (*C*) Lateral radiograph of the TL spine in a dog with underdeveloped accessory processes. (*D*) Dorsal aspect of T12-T13 bone specimen. Arrows identify the well-developed accessory processes on T13 only (accessory processes of T12 are hidden by the cranial process of T13). (*E*) Oblique dorsal lateral view of the T12-T13 bone specimen. With this perspective, the T12 accessory process is also visible.

sequela to caudal articular process dysplasia, has been documented in the pug,[4,14] pug mixes,[14] and other breeds.[5,13] As proposed by Penderis and colleagues,[13] stenotic canal lesions in the basset hound,[16,18] large breed dogs such as the German shepherd dog, Shiloh shepherd,[25] and others[20] may be a variant of articular process dysplasia. Either dysplastic *cranial* articular processes induce the formation of hyperplastic caudal articular processes of the articulating vertebral body or, as pictured in **Fig. 11**, hyperplastic cranial articular processes partially efface the vertebral canal.

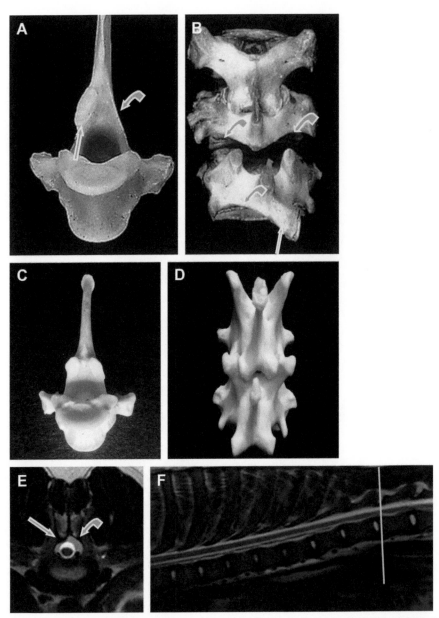

Fig. 9. Images in *A & B* are post mortem specimens of articular facet dysplasia. (*From* Breit S. Osteological and morphometric observations on intervertebral joints in the canine pre-diaphragmatic thoracic spine (Th1±Th9). Vet J 2002;164(3):216–23, with permission.) Straight arrows identify the normal caudal articular process. The curved arrows indicate the missing caudal articular processes. (*A*) Aplasia of right caudal articular surface at T3 seen in a caudal view. (*B*) Bilateral aplasia of T11 and aplasia of left caudal articular surface of T12 seen in a dorsal view. (*C*) Normal bone specimen of T3 for comparison. (*D*) Normal bone specimens of T12-T13 for comparison. (*E*) T2 Axial image of T12 in a 9 MO Rottweiler with normal right caudal articular process and aplastic left caudal articular process. (*F*) T2 sagittal image of the same 9 MO Rottweiler. The straight line delineates the cut line to image the caudal articular process for the axial sequence.

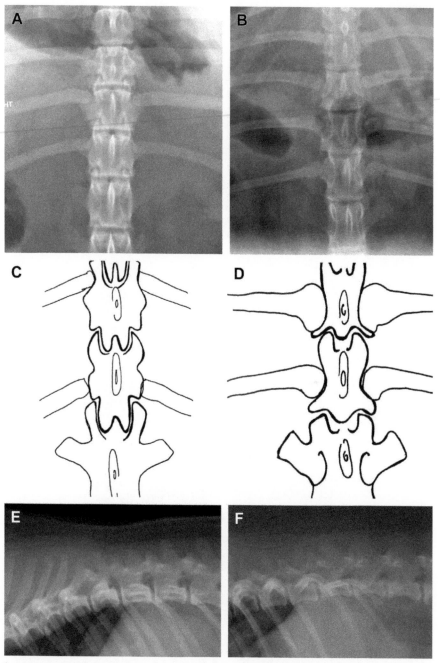

Fig. 10. Dysplastic caudal articular processes can be readily identified on well-positioned and properly exposed radiographs. On the ventrodorsal projection of a normal canine thoracolumbar (TL) spine, the caudal articular process crosses the IVD space and will have a rounded cursive W-shape. In dogs with dysplastic caudal articular processes, the shape is more akin to a broad lowercase "u" shape. (A) VD projection of the TL junction in a normal dog. (B) VD projection of the TL spine in a pug with dysplastic caudal articular processes. (C) Schematic drawing of the rounded cursive W-shape of the normal caudal articular processes. (D) Schematic drawing of the broad lowercase "u" shape of the dysplastic caudal articular processes. (E) Lateral radiograph of the TL spine in a pug with caudal articular process dysplasia of T11-T12. (F) Lateral radiograph of the TL spine in a pug with caudal articular process dysplasia T11-T12 and T12-T13.

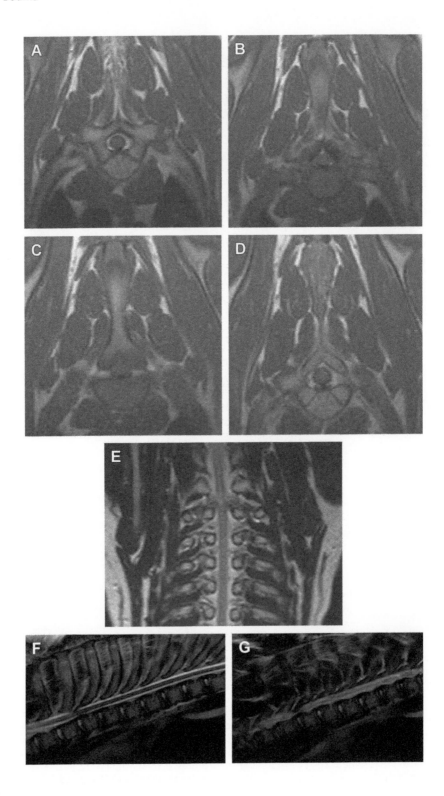

Contrary to previous literature,[3,10] the common theme in more recent publications is the identification of dysplasia of the caudal articular process in the thoracic spine caudal to the diaphragmatic vertebra, T10 (see **Fig. 10**). This important difference touches on the 3 factors as listed previously: location, function, and anatomy. As outlined above, the caudal thoracic spine has smaller diameter and is a transitional portion of the spine. The form and function of the articular processes are dramatically different. The opposing angles of the cranial articular process and caudal articular process of T10 allow for great mobility (see **Fig. 4**). The additional stabilizing factors of the costoverterbral articulations and associated soft tissue structures are absent in the caudal thoracic spine.[1,2] The loss of an articular process in T10 or adjoining vertebra (to the level of L3) can destabilize this segment of the vertebral column. Over time, chronic micromotion can lead to fibrosis, adhesions, tethering of the spinal cord, disruption of normal cerebrospinal fluid (CSF) circulation, possible arachnoid diverticula/cyst formation, and occasionally, gliosis (**Fig. 12**). Clinically, these secondary parenchymal changes of the spinal cord and meninges manifest as slowly progressive constrictive myelopathies.[4,14]

Differentiation between constrictive myelopathy and conditions with similar presenting signs of T3-L3 myelopathy is definitively made with the aid of imaging (survey radiographs + CT ± MRI), although one may be able to accurately predict constrictive myelopathy versus intervertebral disc disease (IVDD) by paying close attention to historical and physical examination findings. Dogs with constrictive myelopathy often do not have signs of pain or discomfort on palpation of the spine, presumably due to the slow, insidiously progressive nature of this abnormality. Urinary and fecal incontinence commonly occur before the development of nonambulatory status.[4]

At the time of this publication, there has been no convincing evidence that caudal articular process dysplasia is a predisposing factor in IVDD.[3,4,10,14] In fact, in cases of IVDD that correspond to locations of caudal articular process, dysplasia may be coincidental.[3,5,14] In a multi-institutional retrospective study of 51 pugs and pug mixes, concurrent IVDD at the site of caudal articular process dysplasia was only 29%. The most common location of IVDD in this group of dogs was T12-T13.[14] The most common location of IVDD in small breed and chondrodystrophic dogs has been reported as T12-T13 in multiple studies.[26–28] Alternatively, in nonchondrodystrophic breeds, extradural spinal cord compression may occur secondary to enlargement of the articulating cranial articular process because of compensatory hypertrophy or degenerative osseous and soft tissue proliferation.[13]

In addition to dysplasia of the caudal articular process identified in the pug,[4,14] pug mixes,[14] and other breeds,[5,13] there may be additional dysplastic conditions of the articular processes that have been previously classified as congenital or developmental stenosis.[11,20,22–25] However, further studies are needed.

◄────────────────────────────────────

Fig. 11. Selected images of an MRI examination of a 4-month-old German shepherd dog with stenosis of the cranial thoracic vertebral canal due to bilateral hypertrophy of the cranial articular processes of T3. (*A*) T1 axial image immediately cranial to the lesion demonstrates the normal dimension of the canal. (*B, C*) T1 axial sequential images through the stenotic canal due to bilateral cranial articular process hypertrophy of T3. (*D*) T1 axial image immediately caudal to the lesion demonstrating the return to normal dimension of the canal. (*E*) T1 coronal image demonstrating the narrowing of the canal due to cranial articular process hypertrophy. (*F, G*) T2 midline and parasagittal images demonstrating the focal stenosis of the canal due to cranial articular process hypertrophy.

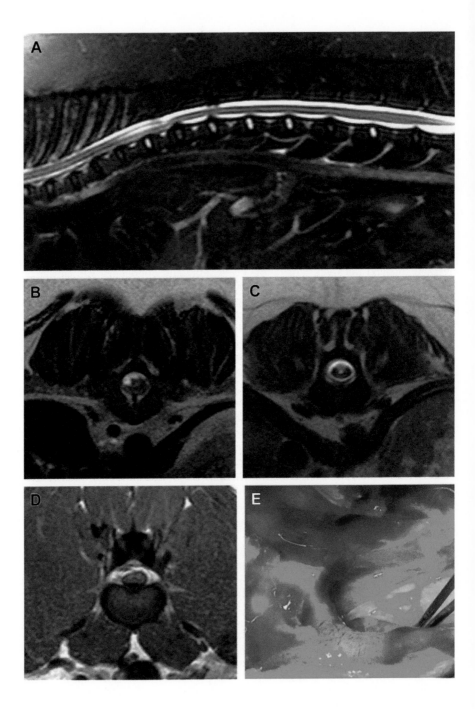

A potential additional manifestation of articular process dysplasia has been documented in the Scottish deerhound. Unlike in those previously mentioned, this occurs in the cranial cervical vertebral column at the level of C2-C3.[23] Kinzel and colleagues[23] defined this specific anomaly "arthrosis of the cervical articular process joints," which they identified in 9 Scottish deerhounds in Germany that had no familial relationship (review limited to 3 generations). Characteristic finding in this series of dogs is enlargement of the articular processes, either unilateral or bilateral. This enlargement was determined to be a degenerative change. The patients in this series ranged in age from 3 to 6 years. The enlargement of the cranial articular process of C3 may be a degenerative change secondary to dysplasia of the caudal articular process of C2, but it may also be possible that this represents a primary hyperplastic dystrophic change of the cranial process of C3; this is an interesting possibility that is another avenue yet to be fully explored.

The clinical impact of cervical arthosis differs from the other articular process anomalies. Although there may be secondary stenosis of the vertebral canal, these patients do not have neurologic dysfunction related to compression of the spinal cord or nerve roots; this is an example of how location can significantly impact the clinical significance. The main presenting sign in these dogs is pain associated with flexion of the neck. As reviewed in the anatomy section, the cranial cervical vertebral canal is large, and therefore, this is not a source of extradural cord compression. The cervical articular process joints have great mobility, and it is easy to understand how an abnormally large process can lead to discomfort. Similar to other articular process anomalies reviewed in this article, cause is undetermined at this time. However, there is strong evidence that this may be a genetic condition.

Caudal articular process dysplasias are congenital anomalies in which the underlying cause has not been identified. Several hypotheses have been suggested for hypoplastic and aplastic caudal articular processes. The first hypothesis postulates that a mutation of the *Hox* gene, which is responsible for the production of Homebox proteins, may cause dysregulation of chondrocyte proliferation and differentiation; this in turn may result in failure of caudal articular processes either to ossify or to form.[4,5] Alternatively, caudal articular fact hypoplasia or aplasia may be associated

---

Fig. 12. This series of images illustrates several of the potential sequelae of caudal articular process dysplasia in the caudal thoracic-cranial lumbar spine. The chronic micromotion can lead to fibrosis, adhesions, tethering of the cord, disruption of normal CSF circulation, and arachnoid diverticula (arachnoid cysts). (*A*) T2 sagittal image of the thoracolumbar spine in a pug with caudal articular process dysplasia in 2 locations (T10-T11 and T12-T13). This image demonstrates abnormal accumulations of dorsal CSF consistent with abnormal CSF circulation and arachnoid diverticula. The increased signal intensity associated with central canal could represent syrinx formation, early gliosis, or both. The hypointensities partially effacing the dorsal CSF signal at T11-T12 may represent either hypertrophy of the soft tissue structures of the articular process joint or adhesions. Axial images are important to further define. (*B*) Axial T2 sequence in a pug with caudal articular process dysplasia. The eccentric accumulation of dorsal right lateral CSF and deformation of the cord shape are consistent with fibrosis and hence tethering of the cord. (*C*) Axial T2 sequence in a pug with caudal articular process dysplasia. The increased signal intensity within the dorsal aspect of the cord is consistent with gliosis. The increased volume of dorsal CSF may represent an early arachnoid diverticula. (*D, E*) Both images are from the same patient with constrictive myelopathy, and the thin hypointense bands crossing the dorsal aspect of the canal in (*D*) correspond to the triangular band of fibrous tissue indicated with the hemostats in this intraoperative photo illustrated in (*E*).

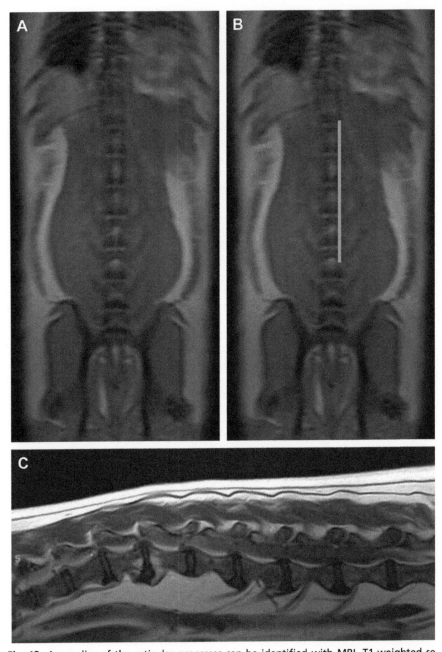

Fig. 13. Anomalies of the articular processes can be identified with MRI. T1-weighted sequences will provide the best image detail of the osseous structures. Attention to detail is imperative. Patient positioning is the first step of imaging the articular processes. Localizer sequence will aid in determining if the spine is in a straight sagittal plane. Placement of the cut lines for the sagittal sequences can be performed on the coronal localizer, T1 or T2 coronal sequence. (*A*) Coronal localizer with straight lumbar spine. (*B*) Coronal localizer with suggested cut line for the sagittal sequence to obtain images of the articular processes. (*C*) T1 sagittal sequence of a pug with caudal articular process dysplasia of T12, T13, and L1.

with dysgenesis of either the 2 neural arch centers.[4,5] Finally, it may be due to failure of accessory ossification center to develop or unite with the lamina.[5]

DIAGNOSTIC IMAGING

As previously mentioned, the availability of cross-sectional imaging such as CT and MRI provides detailed information of both the osseous and the soft tissue structures of the spine that are not possible with planar imaging such as radiography. The utility of survey spinal radiography as a screening tool for congenital spinal anomalies such as articular process dysplasia should not be dismissed (see **Fig. 10**). The astute observer of well-positioned, collimated, and properly exposed orthogonal projections of the spine will be able to better plan for and choose the correct advanced cross-sectional imaging modality if both CT and MRI (**Fig. 13**) are available.

If available facility-wise and financially, the combination of both CT and MRI (in addition to survey radiography) will provide the most information for all articular process anomalies. Detailed information pertaining to osseous abnormalities is best provided by CT. MRI provides superior soft tissue detail of muscle, ligaments, and joint capsules, as well as the spinal cord, spinal nerves/nerve roots, and meninges. If MRI is the only advanced imaging modality available, T1-weighted sequences in all 3 planes with or without contrast (depending on the individual case) are recommended to provide adequate information about the bony skeletal structures.

TREATMENT

In cases of compressive and constrictive myelopathies, surgical decompression and stabilization are often recommended. Stabilization of the affected segment is recommended to decrease micromotion instability to further avoid additional neurologic deterioration. Compressive and restrictive myelopathies may result in irreversible mechanical derangement of nervous tissue with loss of axons, myelin and secondary gliosis, and occasionally, fibrosis.[4]

Medical management should be considered an option in situations in which surgery is not financially available for the owner. The combination of low-dose prednisone and Tramadol or nonsteroidal anti-inflammatory drugs and Tramadol may provide adequate relief of clinical signs. The addition of pregabalin for either combination is recommended if pain relief is not achieved. For more information on medical management options, please see Curtis W. Dewey, Emma Davies and Jennifer L. Bouma: Kyphosis and Kyphoscoliosis Associated with Congenital Malformations of the Thoracic Vertebral Bodies in Dogs, in this issue.

Successful alleviation of pain for most cases of cervical arthrosis described in the Scottish deerhound case series was achieved with an injection of triamcinolone acetonide and lidocaine hydrochloride into the affected articular process joint under fluoroscopic guidance. Fluoroscopic guidance confirms the imaging diagnosis as well as provides relief for the patient.[23]

SUMMARY

Not all congenital articular process anomalies are incidental. The advent of widespread usage of advanced cross-sectional imaging such as CT and MRI allows for more detailed evaluation of the structures of the vertebral column, spinal cord, and nerve roots. Location, normal anatomic variation of the articular processes, and articular process function of the affected segment of the vertebral column are the factors that dictate the clinical relevance as well as clinical manifestation.

Previously, articular process hypoplasia and aplasia had been identified in the pre-diaphragmatic thoracic spine (cranial to T10). The lack of clinical signs associated with these lesions compared with more recently identified lesions in the caudal thoracic and cranial lumbar spine that have clinical significance exemplifies the importance not only of location but also of different functions of the articular processes in particular regions of the vertebral column. The articular processes in the cranial to midthoracic spine primarily aid in weight-bearing and contribute little in terms of stabilizing. In locations of the vertebral column in which articular processes play a larger role in stabilization, such as the more mobile caudal thoracic and cranial lumbar vertebral column, hypoplastic or aplastic processes may result in minimal loss of instability. Over time, chronic micromotion can lead to fibrosis, adhesions, tethering of the cord, disruption of normal CSF circulation, possible arachnoid diverticula ("cyst" formation), and occasionally, gliosis.

Large or giant breed dogs with enlargement of an articular process in portions of the vertebral column where the internal diameter of the canal is large, such as the cranial cervical region, are more likely to manifest as primary pain localized to the articular process and less likely to result in neurologic signs. However, if the same lesion were to occur in a small or chondrodystrophic dog, the presenting complaint is more likely to be neurologic in nature due to similar cord diameter but smaller-diameter vertebral canal. Similarly, patients of any size with enlargement of processes in a segment of the vertebral canal, which is narrower, such as the cranial thoracic region, are more likely to exhibit neurologic signs due to stenosis of the canal.

Articular process dysplasia is a term that encompasses the spectrum of known as well as unknown (potential) congenital articular process anomalies. Although no definitive cause has been identified, breed-specific anomalies that have already been identified are strong indicators of a genetic component.

REFERENCES

1. Evans HE. The skeleton: the vertebral column. In: Evans HE, editor. Miller's anatomy of the dog. 3rd edition. Philadelphia: WB Saunders Co; 1993. p. 166–81.
2. Evans HE. Arthology: ligaments and joints of the vertebral column. In: Evans HE, editor. Miller's anatomy of the dog. 3rd edition. Philadelphia: WB Saunders Co; 1993. p. 225–33.
3. Breit S. Osteological and morphometric observations on intervertebral joints in the canine pre-diaphragmatic thoracic spine (Th1–Th9). Vet J 2002;164(3): 216–23.
4. Fisher SC, Shores A, Simpson ST. Constrictive myelopathy secondary to hypoplasia or aplasia of the thoracolumbar caudal articular processes in Pugs: 11 cases (1993–2009). J Am Vet Med Assoc 2013;242(2):223–9.
5. Werner T, McNicholas WT, Kim J, et al. Aplastic articular processes in a dog with intervertebral disk rupture of the 12th to 13th thoracic vertebral space. J Am Anim Hosp Assoc 2004;40(6):490–4.
6. Smith G, Walter MC. Spinal decompressive procedures and dorsal compartment injuries: comparative biomechanical study in canine cadavers. Am J Vet Res 1988;49(2):266–73.
7. Anderson DM, Keith J, Novak PD, et al. Dorland's illustrated medical dictionary. 29th edition. Philadelphia: WB Saunders Co; 2000.

8. Evans HE. Spinal cord and meninges: spinal cord segments. In: Evans HE, editor. Miller's anatomy of the dog. 3rd edition. Philadelphia: WB Saunders Co; 1993. p. 800–6.

9. Hoerlein BF. Intervertebral disc protrusions in the dog. I. Incidence and pathological lesions. Am J Vet Res 1953;14(51):260–9.

10. Morgan JP. Congenital anomalies of the vertebral column of the dog: a study of the incidence and significance based on a radiographic and morphologic study 1. Vet Radiol 1968;9(1):21–9.

11. Westworth BR, Sturges DK. Congenital spinal malformations in small animals. Vet Clin North Am Small Anim Pract 2010;40(5):951–81.

12. Bailey CS, Morgan JP. Congenital spinal malformations. Vet Clin North Am Small Anim Pract 1992;22(4):985–1015.

13. Penderis J, Schwarz T, McConnell JF, et al. Dysplasia of the caudal vertebral articular processes in four dogs: results of radiographic, myelographic and magnetic resonance imaging investigations. Vet Rec 2005;156(19):601–5.

14. Full A, Dewey CW, Bouma JL. Prevelance and magnetic resonance imaging of intervertebral disc disease in pugs with caudal articular process dysplasia of the thoracolumbar Spine. ACVR Proceedings. St Louis, MO, October 21–24, 2014.

15. Done SH, Drew RA, Robins GM, et al. Hemivertebra in the dog: clinical and pathological observations. Vet Rec 1975;96(14):313–7.

16. Stigen Ø, Hagen G, Kolbjørnsen Ø. Stenosis of the thoracolumbar vertebral canal in a basset hound. J Small Anim Pract 1990;31(12):621–3.

17. Gutierrez-Quintana R, Guevar J, Stalin C, et al. A proposed radiographic classification scheme for congenital thoracic vertebral malformations in brachycephalic "screw-tailed" dog breeds. Vet Radiol Ultrasound 2014; 55(6):585–91.

18. Wright F, Rest JR, Palmer AC. Ataxia of the Great Dane caused by stenosis of the cervical vertebral canal: comparison with similar conditions in the Basset Hound, Doberman Pincher, Ridgeback and thoroughbred horse. J Small Anim Pract 1973;92:1–6.

19. Palmer AC, Wallace ME. Deformation of the cervical vertebrae in basset hounds. Vet Rec 1967;80:430–3.

20. Johnson P, De Risio L, Sparkes A, et al. Clinical, morphologic, and morphometric features of cranial thoracic spinal stenosis in large and giant breed dogs. Vet Radiol Ultrasound 2012;53(5):524–34.

21. Knecht CD, Blevins WE, Raffe MR. Stenosis of the thoracic spinal canal in English Bulldogs. J Am Anim Hosp Assoc 1979;15:181–3.

22. Stalin CE, Pratt JN, Smith PM, et al. Thoracic stenosis causing lateral compression of the spinal cord in two immature Dogues de Bordeaux. Vet Comp Orthop Traumatol 2009;22(1):59–62.

23. Kinzel S, Hein S, Buecker A, et al. Diagnosis and treatment of arthrosis of cervical articular process joints in Scottish Deerhounds: 9 cases (1998-2002). J Am Vet Med Assoc 2003;223(9):1311–5.

24. De Decker S, De Risio L, Lowrie M, et al. Cervical vertebral stenosis associated with a vertebral arch anomaly in the basset hound. J Vet Intern Med 2012;26(6):1374–82.

25. McDonnell JJ, Knowles KE, deLahunta A, et al. Thoracolumbar spinal cord compression due to vertebral process degenerative joint disease in a family of Shiloh Shepherd dogs. J Vet Intern Med 2003;17(4):530–7.

26. Mayhew PD, McLear RC, Ziemer LS, et al. Risk factors for recurrence of clinical signs associated with thoracolumbar intervertebral disk herniation in dogs: 229 cases (1994-2000). J Am Vet Med Assoc 2004;225(8):1231–6.

27. Naudé SH, Lambrechts NE, Wagner WM. Association of preoperative magnetic resonance imaging findings with surgical features in Dachshunds with thoracolumbar intervertebral disk extrusion. J Am Vet Med Assoc 2008;232(5):702–8.
28. Brisson BA. Intervertebral disc disease in dogs. Vet Clin North Am Small Anim Pract 2010;40(5):829–58.

Spina Bifida, Meningomyelocele, and Meningocele

Rachel B. Song, VMD, MS[a], Eric N. Glass, DVM, MS[a],
Marc Kent, DVM[b],*

KEYWORDS

- Congenital malformation • Meningocele • Meningomyelocele • Neural tube defect
- Spina bifida

KEY POINTS

- The cause of spina bifida with or without meningomyelocele or meningocele (MC) is likely related to genetic and environmental factors.
- Spina bifida with or without meningomyelocele or MC can be associated with other congenital abnormalities of the vertebrae, central nervous system (CNS), and adjacent soft tissues.
- A thorough physical and neurologic examination is warranted in all animals in which an anomaly is suspected.
- Consideration should be given to imaging the entire CNS and adjacent structures to identify coexistent malformations.
- Surgical interventions may be considered in select animals to potentially prevent worsening of signs. In some cases, neurologic improvement may also occur.

INTRODUCTION

Neural tube defects (NTD) are a collection of congenital malformations that typically occur as a result of abnormal development and/or closure of the neural tube during embryogenesis. Development of the central nervous system (CNS) is a precisely timed and highly regulated process that is integrated intimately with the development of the vertebrae, paravertebral musculature, and overlying skin, in addition to other structures such as the distal gastrointestinal and urinary tracts. Consequently, whereas the term NTD connotes anomalous development of the CNS, more broadly, NTDs

The authors have nothing to disclose.
[a] Department of Neurology and Neurosurgery, Red Bank Veterinary Hospital, 197 Hance Avenue, Tinton Falls, NJ 07724, USA; [b] Department of Small Animal Medicine & Surgery, College of Veterinary Medicine, University of Georgia, 2200 College Station Road, Athens, GA 30602, USA
* Corresponding author.
E-mail address: mkent1@uga.edu

Vet Clin Small Anim 46 (2016) 327–345
http://dx.doi.org/10.1016/j.cvsm.2015.10.007
0195-5616/16/$ – see front matter Published by Elsevier Inc.

encompass anomalous development of the vertebrae, paravertebral muscles, and skin in addition to the CNS, and implies the possible coexistence of anomalous development of other anatomic structures. NTDs can be further classified based on whether they are open, exposed neural tissues and leaking cerebrospinal fluid (CSF), or closed, not exposed neural tissues and not leaking CSF.

The terminology used in the literature to describe NTDs is often nonspecific, confusing, or inconsistently applied. **Table 1** contains common terms and their definitions. In particular, several terms are used synonymously with NTD, including spina bifida and spinal dysraphism. Spina bifida is the most commonly used term to describe NTD. Strictly speaking, spina bifida is the embryologic failure of fusion of 1 or more vertebral arches (laminae); subtypes of spina bifida are based on the degree and pattern of malformation associated with neuroectoderm involvement.[1] It can be qualified as aperta (open), cystica (closed), or occulta (hidden or have a concealed external demarcation). Spina bifida alone may not be associated with clinical signs; however, it may be accompanied with spinal cord malformation. The Greek origin of the term *raphe* means the line of union of 2 contiguous bilaterally symmetric structures.[1] In the context of the neural tube, there is an implication of a lack of fusion along the midline of the neural tube.[1] Although terms such as spina bifida and dysraphism are often used in the literature interchangeably, the more broad term NTD may be preferable. Where possible, the authors have tried to use the term NTD to not only encompass spinal cord malformations and vertebral malformations, but also to focus attention on a common pathophysiologic basis notable for neural tube development.

The most common NTDs in humans include spina bifida and anencephaly.[11,12] The cause of NTDs is multifaceted, with contributions from a varying combination of genetic predispositions and environmental interactions. Human estimates for the prevalence of spina bifida in the United States are currently 3.39 per 10,000 live births.[11,13] NTDs in domestic animals are likely underreported with reports limited to single cases and small case series. Although the current prevalence in dogs and cats is unknown, previous reports suggest a prevalence of spina bifida of 0.006% in dogs and 0.09% in cats.[14]

NTDs can occur anywhere along the vertebral column although the majority of reported spina bifida and associated meningomyelocele (MMC) or meningocele (MC) cases occur within the lumbosacral spinal cord and vertebral column. Animals with lumbosacral NTDs display characteristic physical, neurologic, and diagnostic findings. Early recognition of NTDs may allow for improved outcomes for affected animals. The goal of this article is to provide a summary of the embryology and the proposed mechanisms for the congenital defects, outline the clinical signs, diagnostic findings and treatment options that are available for dogs and cats today.

EMBRYOLOGY

The development of the CNS is initiated with the formation of the neuroectoderm, which is derived from proliferative epithelial cells of the ectoderm germ layer. During primary neurulation, the neuroectoderm (neural plate) elongates and bends at the medial hinge point at the ventral most aspect of the neural plate. The medial hinge point remains anchored to the notochord along the long axis of the developing embryo. The notochord provides important signaling molecules such as *sonic hedgehog* for the formation of the ventral spinal cord. The notochord eventually becomes the nucleus pulposus of the intervertebral discs. The lateral margins (neural folds) of the neural plate then elevate until they fuse dorsally, creating a central neural groove and eventually the neural tube[3,5,15–17] (**Fig. 1**). Under the influence of signaling

Table 1
Selected nomenclature used in classification of neural tube defects

Term	Definition	Comments
Meningocele (MC)	Protrusion of meninges through open vertebral arch or cranial bones	—
Meningomyelocele (MMC)	Protrusion of meninges and nervous tissue through open vertebral arch	—
Meningoencephalocele (MEC)	Protrusion of meninges and brain tissue through defect in cranial bones	Further classified depending on the cranial bone defect (occipital, frontoethmoidal, basal, cranial vault)[2]
Myelodysplasia	Any malformation of the spinal cord owing to abnormal interaction of the notochord, paraxial mesoderm, and neural plate during neurulation[3]	—
Spinal cord dysraphism	Failure of the neural folds to appose and close, resulting in failed neural tube closure[3]	"Weimaraner spinal dysraphism" owing to a frameshift mutation in the NKX2-8 gene is considered a misnomer and is more accurately described as myelodysplasia[4]
Myeloschisis	Failure of neural tube closure resulting in persistent attachment of the cutaneous ectoderm to the neural plate and inability of the vertebral arches to close around the open neural plate[5]	Always results in spina bifida
Dermal sinus tract	Failed separation of the neural tube from the skin ectoderm causing tubular sacs lined with hair follicles, sweat, and sebaceous glands that typically extends from the dorsal midline to underlying tissues	Types I–V depending on the ventral extent of the tubular sacs[6,7] Duplication of FGF3, FGF4, FGF19, and ORAOV1 gene mutations responsible for the dorsal hair ridge in Rhodesian and Thai Ridgeback dogs predisposes these breeds[8] Differs from dermoid cysts, which are closed epithelium-lined sacs with liquefied substance[9] Differs from pilonidal cysts, which are acquired secondary to foreign bodies, such as hair[6]
Spina bifida	Failure of the vertebral arch(es) to close over the spinal cord	May be associated with MC or MMC The terms occulta (no neural tissue involved), cystica/manifesta/aperta (associated MC or MMC through vertebral defect) are used depending on the amount of neural and associated tissue involvement[10]

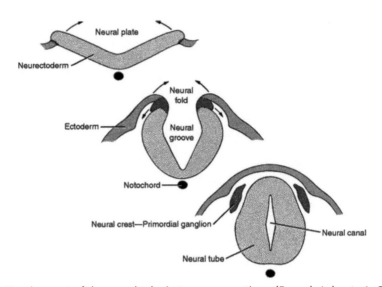

Fig. 1. Development of the neural tube in transverse sections. (*From* de Lahunta A, Glass E, Kent M. Development of the nervous system: malformation. In: de Lahunta A, Glass E, Kent M, editors. Veterinary neuroanatomy and clinical neurology. 4th edition. Saunders; 2015. p. 46; with permission.)

molecules such as *bone morphogenetic protein* from the surface ectodermal cells, bilateral columns of neural crest cells form at the juncture of neural and nonneural ectoderm. The neural crest cells contribute to the formation of the spinal ganglia and the dorsal spinal cord (**Fig. 2**). Neural tube fusion occurs at multiple sites that vary in location and number depending on the species[5,12,15,17–19] (**Figs. 3** and **4**). From the points of fusion, neural tube closure proceeds in an unidirection or bidirection, depending on the point of fusion and species. The neural tube eventually separates from the surface ectoderm mediated through expression of different cell adhesion molecules.

The caudal most aspect of the neural tube undergoes secondary neurulation, or cavitation. In this region, a column of neuroepithelial cells, caudal cell mass, extends caudally from the neural tube on midline, ventral to the ectoderm. Cavitation of the column of cells creates the central lumen that is continuous with the neural tube created during primary neurulation.

PATHOGENESIS

Failure of proper closure of the neural tube can lead to NTDs anywhere along the neural axis. When the rostral neuropore fails to close, NTDs affecting the brain and skull such as cranioschisis with or without MC or MECs may occur. If the neural tissue comes in direct contact with amniotic fluid, degeneration of previously developed neural tissue occurs.[19] If this occurs in the brain, anencephaly ensues, which is invariably fatal; in the spinal cord, animals may survive with variable degrees of morbidity and mortality depending on the severity of the defect.

Within the vertebral column, NTDs at the level of the lumbosacral vertebral column are most commonly encountered in practice. At this level, NTDs may occur owing to errors during primary neurulation, although errors of secondary neurulation have also been suggested.[3,15,20,21] However, even if such NTDs are initially the result of a

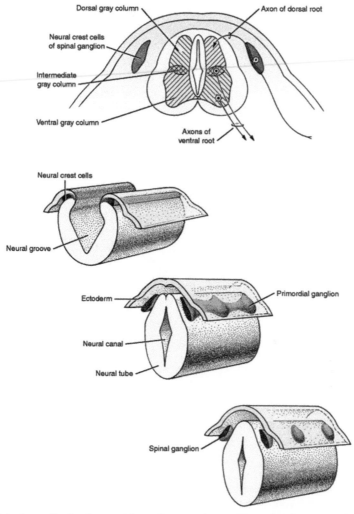

Fig. 2. Spinal ganglia development from the neural crest. (*From* de Lahunta A, Glass E, Kent M. Development of the nervous system: malformation. In: de Lahunta A, Glass E, Kent M, editors. Veterinary neuroanatomy and clinical neurology. 4th edition. Saunders; 2015. p. 51; with permission.)

disturbance of primary neurulation and a persistently open caudal neuropore, ensuing errors in secondary neurulation are also likely to occur.[20] Experimental studies in the curly-tail mutant mice, a well-established model for human NTD, has also suggested that an imbalance in dorsoventral cell proliferation, leading to excessive ventral curvature of embryo and stresses on the neural tube, leading to delay or cessation of the closure of the caudal neuropore.[15] Similarly, animal species that have less of an axial curvature experience faster closure rates of the caudal neuropore than species with a greater curvature.[17]

In addition to the neural tube failing to close, a reopening of an already closed neural tube (ie, owing to excessive CSF production or increased CSF pressure) has also been suggested. This may account for defects occur later in development, or over an

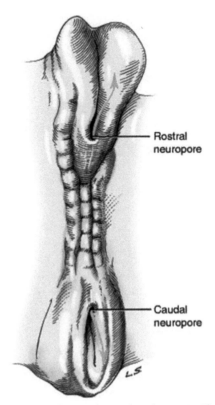

Rostral
neuropore

Caudal
neuropore

Fig. 3. Dorsal view of neural tube closure. (*From* de Lahunta A, Glass E, Kent M. Development of the nervous system: malformation. In: de Lahunta A, Glass E, Kent M, editors. Veterinary neuroanatomy and clinical neurology. 4th edition. Saunders; 2015. p. 46; with permission.)

extended period of time during gestation, rather than during the stages of primary and secondary neurulation.[17,21] Hyperplastic dorsal neural tube cells preventing fusion of the neural tube, or vascular disturbance causing ischemic damage to the dorsal vertebral column, have also been suggested.[14,22–25]

ETIOLOGY

The cause of NTDs is likely multifaceted. A threshold model, where multiple genetic and environmental variants interact to cause such NTD, has been suggested.[4] Given the overrepresentation in certain breeds of dogs and cats, human families, and ethnicities, genetics likely plays an important role. More than 200 gene mutations involved in important biological pathways, such as folate metabolism and transport, DNA repair, retinoic acid receptors, and planar cell polarity signaling network, have been shown to cause NTDs in mouse models.[4,26,27] Recent whole genome linkage analysis for NTDs showed strong linkage to chromosome 9 arising within a single human family.[27] Another recent study found a small proportion of human patients with spina bifida with a missense mutation in the *NKX2-8* gene, the causative gene for "Weimaraner spinal cord dysraphism," a form of myelodysplasia recognized in that breed.[4]

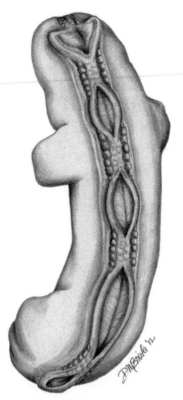

Fig. 4. Proposed multiple site closure of neural tube during neurulation. (*From* Song RB, Glass EN, Kent M, et al. Surgical correction of a sacral meningomyelocele in a dog. J Am Anim Hosp Assoc 2014;50:441; with permission.)

Monozygomatic twinning and other single gene disorders in humans have also been associated with increased risk of NTDs.[17,26]

In humans, folic acid supplementation by a mother before completion of neural tube formation of the fetus at 28 days of gestation has reduced significantly congenital NTDs. The evidence was so unequivocal that the US Food and Drug Administration mandated the addition of folic acid to grain products in 1998, with many other countries following suit thereafter.[1,12,26,28] In humans, other diseases of the mother during pregnancy such as diabetes mellitus, obesity, vitamin B_{12} deficiency, choline deficiency, and exposure to medications such as valproic acid and carbamazepine also are associated with NTDs.[12,13,15,29] Therefore, improving access to health care, prenatal supplements, and continuing the trend toward folic acid fortification worldwide are important human public health concerns that should result in decreasing the rates of preventable NTDs.

In experimental studies of cats, the administration of drugs to a pregnant queen, such as the antifungal agents griseofulvin[30] and ethylenethiourea,[31] and toxic agents such as methylmercury[32] and hydroxyurea,[31] has been associated with increased congenital malformations of kittens, including NTDs like cranium bifidum, spina bifida, and absent caudal vertebrae.[30] Given the rapid mitoses that neuropithelial cells undergo during neurulation, it is not surprising that medications that interfere with cell division are associated with congenital defects.

PATHOLOGIC FINDINGS

As mentioned, spina bifida is a failure of the neural arches to close dorsal to the spinal cord. Alone, this does not result in clinical signs. In instances in which there is a concurrent MC, there is protrusion of the meninges, through the opening in the laminae and into midline of the epaxial muscles (**Fig. 5**). The protruding meninges may extend dorsal to connect to the skin but remain as a closed, blind ending sac or it may remain "open" at the skin and leak CSF (**Figs. 6 and 7**). With MMC, there are neural tissues that course in the MC (**Fig. 8**).

DIAGNOSIS
Signalment

Moderate to severe forms of NTD, such as spina bifida and MMC or MC, are typically diagnosed in young animals. Although a congenital anomaly can be seen in any breed, certain breeds have been overrepresented with spina bifida and other vertebral anomalies being more prevalent the English Bulldogs[14,21,23,24,33] and the German shepherd dogs.[18,25] In cats, the most notable breed is the Manx, characterized by sacrocaudal dysgenesis resulting in a high incidence of spina bifida and MMC[34–37] (**Figs. 9 and 10**). This trait is secondary to an autosomal-dominant trait, resulting in phenotypic morphology such as "rumpies" (absent caudal vertebrae), "rumpy risers" (several caudal vertebrae), "stumpies" (several mobile caudal vertebrae), or "longies" (normal tail).[37,38] Although clinically normal, the stumpies differ from tailed cats in the length of the tail, caudal nerves, and filum terminale.[37] In contrast, rumpies are more likely to display an abnormal gait, incontinence, an abnormal sacrum with absent caudal vertebrae, and various degrees of spina bifida, tethering of the spinal cord, MC, and MMC.[37] It is unfortunate that the current breed standards for the Manx cat include complete taillessness, which encourages for selection of rumpies, leading to the persistent breeding of neurologically affected animals.[39] It is also likely that most affected kittens are culled at birth or lost in utero because the homozygous Manx trait is lethal.[38]

Clinical Signs

In animals with less dramatic malformations in which there is no involvement of neural structures, the animal will likely have normal neurologic function. In these cases,

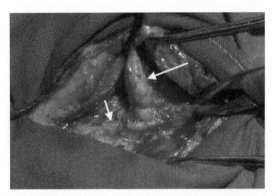

Fig. 5. Intraoperative image of a meningocele. The epaxial muscles have been elevated from the lumbar vertebral column and retracted laterally. A blind ending sac was resected free from its attachment at the skin and dissected ventrally to its connection with the dura mater (*large arrow*). Cranial to the meningocele, the normal dura mater is visible (*small arrow*). Cranial is to the left of the image.

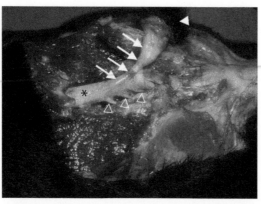

Fig. 6. Gross image at autopsy of a dog with a meningocele. A laminectomy has been performed to allow visualization of the caudal aspect of the lumbar spinal cord (*asterisk*). The meningocele (*large arrows*) extends from the dura mater dorsally to the skin (*arrowhead*). Cranial is to the left of the image.

vertebral column abnormalities such as spina bifida may be found incidentally on radiographs. With increasing severity and complexity of the NTD, affected animals typically present to a veterinarian for evaluation from birth to 8 months of age. Changes in the hair coat and skin associated with a defect on the dorsal midline can be seen (**Figs. 11** and **12**). Dorsal midline cutaneous defects include abnormal streaming of the hair, externally visible depressions where the neuroectoderm failed to separate from the ectoderm, and crusting cutaneous lesions associated with drainage of the CSF to the skin. In cases where the subarachnoid space is continuous with the environment, chronic loss of CSF potentially may lead to hyponatremia and hypochloremia. Surgical correction of the meningocutaneous tract may provide long-term control of electrolytes, although neurologic dysfunction may persist.[35] Meningomyelitis owing to contamination with environmental microorganisms (ostensibly bacteria) may also occur in the presence of a meningocutaneous tract.[36]

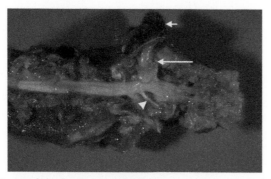

Fig. 7. Gross specimen of the lumbar vertebral column and sacrum. A dorsal laminectomy has been performed and the dura mater has been left intact. There is protrusion of the meninges of the caudal end of the dural sac (*long arrow*), which courses as a "stalk" of blind ending meninges dorsally to attach to the skin (*small arrow*). A sacral spinal nerve (S1) is visible (*arrowhead*). Cranial is to the left of the image.

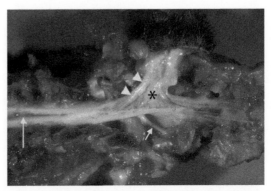

Fig. 8. Same specimen as in **Fig. 7**. A durotomy has been performed. The durotomy has been continued dorsally to open the meningomyelocele (*asterisk*). Neural tissue coursing in the protruded meninges is visualized (*arrowheads*). Cranially, the spinal cord has been incised longitudinally allowing visualization of concurrent syringomyelia (*long arrow*). A sacral spinal nerve (S1) is visible (*short arrow*). Cranial is to the left of the image.

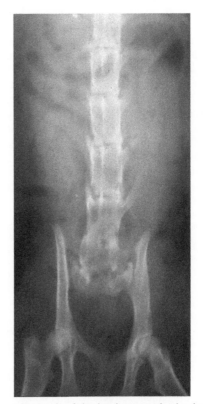

Fig. 9. Ventrodorsal view radiograph of the lumbar vertebral column and pelvis of a Manx cat. There is malformation of L7 with only partial development of the sacrum. Only the cranial aspect of the sacrum is present, the caudal portion of the sacrum and caudal vertebrae are absent.

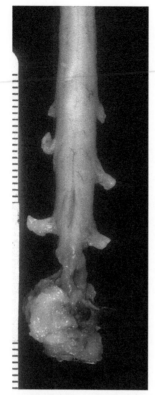

Fig. 10. Gross specimen of the lumbar spinal cord of the cat in **Fig. 9**. The lumbar intumescence and associated nerve roots (which have been transected) seem to be normal. However, the conus medullaris, its roots, and the spinal nerves of the cauda equina are absent.

The majority of NTDs affect the lumbosacral vertebrae, although anomalies can occur focally anywhere along the vertebral column. Additionally, extensive spina bifida involving multiple vertebrae can occur. Depending on the area of the spinal cord involved, varying degrees of general proprioceptive ataxia and upper motor neuron paraparesis or tetraparesis may be seen. When the anomaly occurs at the cervical or lumbar intumescence or affects the associated the roots and spinal nerves, varying degrees of lower motor neuron paresis may be observed. When the lumbar intumescence, its roots, and/or spinal nerves are affected, the animals may display a gait in which both pelvic limbs are advanced simultaneously, referred to as a "bunny hopping" gait.[5] With lesions involving the sacral and caudal nerves, the gait may be normal and signs consist of urinary and/or fecal incontinence, hypalgesia of the overlying skin of the caudal thigh region, genitals, perineum, and tail, as well as protrusion of the penis and decreased or absent tail tone.

Tethered cord syndrome, a syndrome in which excessive stretching and tension on neural tissues occurs owing to abnormal attachments to the vertebrae or skin, may occur in conjunction with MMC and spina bifida,[21,33,36,37] although it may also occur in isolation[40] owing to failure of the neuroectoderm to separate from the ectoderm. As a consequence of the abnormal attachments of the neural tissues in NTD, the disproportionate growth of the vertebral column during skeletal maturation in comparison with the neural tissues causes tension on the spinal cord, roots, and/or spinal

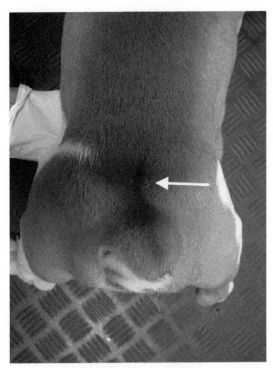

Fig. 11. A dorsal view of the hindend of a 6-month-old English Bulldog that was presented for urinary and fecal incontinence. The hair on the dorsal midline has an abnormal appearance (*arrow*). At that site, there is a palpable indentation of the epaxial muscles. Radiographically, spina bifida was present. Given the neurologic deficits, meningomyelocele was presumed.

nerves, which may result in progressive worsening of neurologic deficits referable to the lumbar intumescence, conus medullaris, and cauda equina. Thus, patients with tethered cord syndrome in conjunction with spina bifida or MMC typically experience progressive worsening of neurologic deficits, such as pelvic limb paresis and varying degrees of fecal and urinary incontinence with skeletal growth.

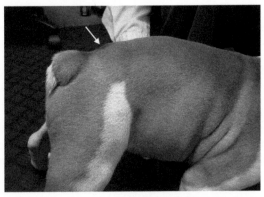

Fig. 12. Lateral view of the same dog in Fig. 11, the dorsal abnormal hair pattern and abrupt change, "dimple" or indentation in the midline is visible (*arrow*).

Finally, it is important to recognize that NTDs may also occur with other congenital abnormalities within the same individual. Therefore, the observation of 1 malformation should prompt careful assessment of the animal for additional anomalies. Congenital abnormalities in dogs and cats observed in association or coexistent with NTDs include hydrocephalus,[14,21,23] arthrogryposis,[14,22,25] syringomyelia,[14,41] cryptorchidism,[18] and a cleft palate.[42]

Imaging

Definitive diagnosis and characterization of NTDs is made with cross-sectional imaging, primarily MRI. Other imaging modalities also may provide some diagnostic information. Apparent anomalous changes to the vertebrae on radiographs include bifid spinous processes of 1 or more vertebrae or an absent spinous process(es)[14,21–24,33,34,41] (**Figs. 13–15**). Importantly, clinically silent, bifid spinous processes may be seen in other vertebrae unassociated with a clinically relevant NTD, such as MMC. Therefore, caution should be exercised when ascribing clinical significance to vertebral anomalies observed on radiographs.

Myelography can be used to evaluate the size and location of the subarachnoid space. With MMCs, myelography typically reveals a widened subarachnoid space that deviates dorsally, extending into the soft tissues outside of the vertebral canal.[7,21,23–25,33,34] Myelography may be performed through the abnormal soft tissue present on the dorsal cutaneous surface of the affected animal.[22] Despite the potential ease in injecting iodinated contrast medium to fill the subarachnoid space, this technique is not recommended because of the possibility of introducing infection into the subarachnoid space.[22] In particular, myelography should be avoided in cases of overt CSF drainage onto the overlying skin to prevent further introduction, or even spread of bacteria to the subarachnoid space and CNS. If myelography is to be performed, injection of contrast medium into the cerebellomedullary cistern should be considered to avoid potentially catastrophic outcomes. Ultimately, the clinician should be aware of the risks of myelography, including seizures, worsening of neurologic signs, and the potential spread of meningomyelitis.

Computed tomography, alone or combined with myelography, provides additional information about the vertebral anomalies and associated neural tissues involved.[7] Tethering of the spinal cord, communication of the dura with an overlying skin depression, and residual nerves and nerve roots may also be visualized.

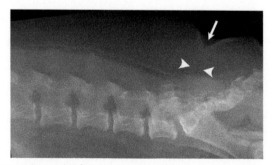

Fig. 13. Lateral view radiograph of the lumbar, sacral, and caudal vertebrae of a 5-month-old English bulldog. There is a "dimple" or indentation where a presumed connection exists between the skin and meningocele (*arrow*). Extending from the skin margin ventrally toward the vertebral column is an increased opacity that likely represents a meningocele (between the *arrowheads*). There is also malformation of the laminae of the sacrum.

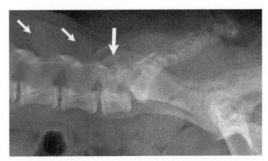

Fig. 14. A lateral view radiograph of the vertebral column from the L5, sacrum, and caudal vertebrae of a 4.5-month-old Bulldog presenting for evaluation of urinary and fecal incontinence. Neurologic examination revealed an easily expressed bladder, absent anal sphincter tone, and analgesia to the skin of the perineum. The spinous processes of L5 and L6 are present (*small arrows*); however, the spinous process of L7 is absent, suggestive of spina bifida (*large arrow*).

Ultrasonography of the affected region may also enable visualization of an MMC.[36] However, ultrasonography is unlikely to provide enough anatomic detail for a specific diagnosis.

Ultimately, MRI is the superior imaging modality to evaluate the vertebral column and associated neural tissues. In addition to precise anatomic detail of MC and MMC, changes involving the spinal cord consistent with syringomyelia, edema, meningitis, and/or gliosis may be observed. MRI can reveal T1-weighted hypointense and T2-weighted hyperintense, fluid-filled space indicative of an MC dorsal to the affected vertebral segments and contiguous with the subarachnoid space via a defect in the lamina of the affected vertebrae[43] (**Figs. 16** and **17**). Spinal cord and nerves extending through the subcutaneous tissues dorsally, indicative of an MMC, may be seen on MRI

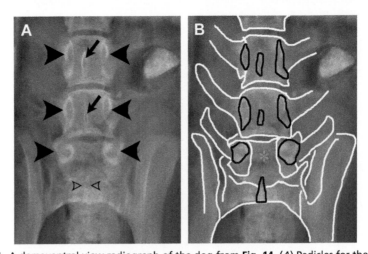

Fig. 15. A dorsoventral view radiograph of the dog from **Fig. 14.** (*A*) Pedicles for the L5, L6, and L7 vertebrae are visible (*large arrowheads*). The spinous processes of the L5 and L6 vertebrae are visible (*small arrows*). The median sacral crest is also visible (between the open *arrowheads*). There is no visible spinous process of L7. (*B*) The edges of the vertebrae and pelvis are outlined in white. The pedicles, spinous processes, and median sacral crest are outlined in black. The L7 spinous process should be present in the region of the asterisk.

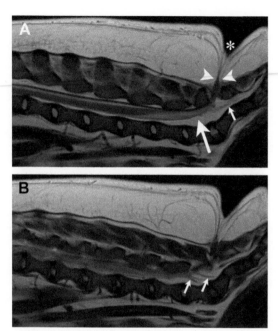

Fig. 16. (*A*) A T2-weighted midline sagittal image of the lumbosacral vertebral column from the dog in **Fig. 13**. The "dimple" or indentation of the skin is visible (*asterisk*). There is meninges, which exit the vertebral column dorsally between the L7 and sacral laminae and connect to the skin (between the *arrowheads*). Notice the dorsal deviation of the spinal dura mater filaments (*large arrow*). (*B*) In a sagittal image just lateral to midline, the nerve roots are visible coursing toward their foramina (*arrows*).

as well.[18] Intravenous contrast administration can also reveal mild contrast enhancement of the abnormal region.

Cerebrospinal Fluid

Although analysis of CSF is unlikely to aide in the diagnosis, in animals with signs or other clinicopathologic data suggestive of an inflammatory response, CSF analysis may be warranted. However, in most animals, CSF analysis is typically normal.[14,22] In animals with patent communication of MC or MMC with the skin surface, CSF analysis may help to identify bacterial contamination of the CSF. In such cases, an aliquot of CSF should be submitted for culture and sensitivity.

THERAPY
Medical Management

In animals with occult spina bifida or a nonpatent meningocutaneous tract that lacks neurologic deficits, specific therapy is not warranted. However, the animal should be monitored during the first few years of life for any neurologic decline that may occur owing to tethered cord syndrome. In cases of MC or MMC with a patent meningocutaneous tract that is allowing CSF to drain, medical management can be considered, by keeping the cutaneous lesion clean.[44] Antiinflammatory medications and antibiotics may be considered. In humans, mild trauma, such as a fall, can cause an exacerbation of CSF leakage from the cutaneous wound.[44] Patients considering medical management are at risk for future worsening and irreversible neurologic sequelae

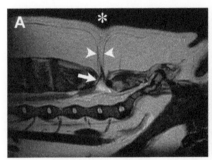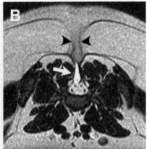

Fig. 17. A T2-weighted sagittal (*A*) and a transverse image (*B*) of the lumbar vertebral column of a 10-month-old FS English Bulldog presenting for urinary and fecal incontinence. Neurologic examination revealed decreased anal sphincter tone and analgesia to the skin of the perineum. There was a palpable "dimple" or indentation of the skin in the caudal lumbar region (*asterisk*). There also was a focal T2-weighted hyperintense region in dorsal region of the vertebral foramen at the L7–sacrum articulation (*large arrow*). This hyperintensity was contiguous with the dura and dorsally extended through a defect in the L7 vertebral arch (*arrowheads*) into the soft tissues to the skin. A tethering of the dura mater was relieved at surgery. The urinary and fecal incontinence improved gradually, then resolved within 5 months of surgery. (*B*) On the transverse T2-weighted image, the T2 hyperintensity consistent with a meningocele is seen extending through the dorsal lamina of L7 (*arrow*) with extension to the skin surface (*arrowheads*).

such as urinary and fecal incontinence, cystitis, urinary tract infections, meningitis, and sensorimotor deficits, requiring further care.

Surgery

Surgical exploration should be strongly considered in cases where there is continuous leakage of CSF to the cutaneous surface, which puts the animal at risk for electrolyte imbalance and meningomyelitis. Similarly, surgical exploration should be considered in those animals for which there is a definitive diagnosis of tethered cord syndrome.

In affected children, early closure of an MMC within 48 hours of delivery is advocated, because delayed surgical closure beyond 72 hours is associated with complications such as meningitis, ventriculitis, and hydrocephalus.[44] Moreover, clinically significant ventriculomegaly, which necessitates life-long shunting, occurs in 80% to 90% of children with MMC even after successful surgery.[45] In fact, despite extensive surgical and medical interventions, the leading cause of death in affected infants is Chiari type II.[46]

Given the paucity of veterinary literature related to surgical intervention, clearly defined surgical procedures for affected animals are lacking. Despite this, it is reasonable to consider pursuing analogous surgical procedures in affected animals. For humans, a durotomy is typically required to free the protruded meninges and neural tissues. Utmost caution is taken to preserve as much neural tissue as possible, but a myelotomy or radiculotomy may be necessary to relieve abnormal attachments, which may result in tension on the spinal cord and nerves in the future. A variety of techniques, including primary closure, exogenous graft materials, and various fascial graft techniques, are used in humans to close dural defects.[1] Similar techniques have been used in animals. However, exogenous graft materials may not be necessary.[18] In the end, the goal of surgery remains to prevent future neurologic deterioration, close any open communications between an MC or MMC and the skin to prevent infection, and if possible to improve neurologic function. The latter is less likely obtainable, however; some affected animals do experience improvement of urinary and/or fecal incontinence.[18] More commonly, affected animals continue to have persistent incontinence, with or without transient worsening perioperatively.[7,21,33]

In humans, postoperative tethered cord syndrome ("spinal cord retethering") owing to scar tissue, silk suture material and dural grafts several years after the initial reparative surgery for MMC has been reported.[47] Although not yet reported in animals, as our veterinary experience in this arena develops, it is likely that similar postoperative complications and sequelae will be recognized.

In the future, it is possible that, as our diagnostic tools and therapeutic interventions improve, in utero diagnosis and surgical interventions may become possible. For affected children, improved prenatal diagnostic tools have led to the ability to diagnose spina bifida and MMC as early as the first trimester.[48] A recent randomized, prospective trial suggested that prenatal surgery to close MMCs before 26 weeks of gestation may lead to improved outcomes when compared with postnatal surgical closure of MMC.[49] A large animal experimental model developed in sheep has provided similar results suggesting the uterine environment (amniotic fluid, trauma, etc) may play a significant role in secondary destruction of exposed neural tissues.[12,48] Although fetal surgery is unlikely to play an important role in veterinary medicine, it poses an interesting opportunity for translational research to broaden our knowledge on the pathogenesis of NTDs across species.

Breeding

It is important that breeders of domestic animals, especially those that are predisposed to NTDs, learn to recognize congenital malformations and practice responsible breeding. For example, the continued selection of tail-lessness in the Manx cat leads to the creation of animals with severe congenital malformations and neurologic deficits that are either incompatible with life, or are unacceptable as a pet. Such breeding practices that lead to such unacceptably high rates of morbidity and mortality cannot, and should not, be condoned. Veterinarians should play a large role in client education to eliminate NTDs where genetics clearly have led to predictable anomalies.

REFERENCES

1. McComb JG. A practical clinical classification of spinal neural tube defects. Childs Nerv Syst 2015;10:1641–57.
2. Martlé VA, Caemaert J, Tshamala M, et al. Surgical treatment of a canine intranasal meningoencephalocele. Vet Surg 2009;38:515–9.
3. Noden DM, de Lahunta A. The embryology of domestic animals: developmental mechanisms and malformations. Baltimore (MD): Williams & Wilkins; 1985.
4. Safra N, Bassuk AG, Ferguson PJ, et al. Genome-wide association mapping in dogs enables identification of the homeobox gene, NKX2-8, as a genetic component of neural tube defects in humans. PLoS Genet 2013;9:e1003646.
5. de Lahunta A, Glass EN, Kent M. Veterinary neuroanatomy and clinical neurology. 4th edition. St Louis (MO): Saunders Elsevier; 2015.
6. Westworth DR, Sturges BK. Congenital spinal malformations in small animals. Vet Clin Small Anim 2010;40:951–81.
7. Ployart S, Doran I, Bomassi E, et al. Myelomeningocoele and a dermoid sinus-like lesion in a French bulldog. Can Vet J 2013;54:1133–6.
8. Salmon Hillbertz NH, Isaksson M, Karlsson EF, et al. Duplication of FGF3, FGF4, FGF19 and ORAOV1 causes hair ridge and predisposition to dermoid sinus in Ridgeback dogs. Nat Genet 2007;39:1318–20.

9. Hillbertz NH. Inheritance of dermoid sinus in the Rhodesian ridgeback. J Small Anim Pract 2005;46:71–4.
10. Lavely JA. Pediatric neurology of the dog and cat. Vet Clin Small Anim 2006;36: 475–501.
11. Boulet SL, Yang Q, Mai C, et al. Trends in the postfortification prevalence of spina bifida and anencephaly in the United State. Birth Defects Res A Clin Mol Teratol 2008;82:527–32.
12. Botto LD, Moore CA, Khoury MJ, et al. Neural-tube defects. N Engl J Med 1999; 341:1509–19.
13. Flores AL, Vellozzi C, Valencia D, et al. Global burden of neural tube defects, risk factors, and prevention. Indian J Community Health 2014;26(Suppl S1):03–5.
14. Wilson JW, Kurtz HJ, Leipold HW, et al. Spina bifida in the dog. Vet Pathol 1979; 16:165–79.
15. Finnell RH, Gould A, Spiegelstein O. Pathobiology and genetics of neural tube defects. Epilepsia 2003;44:14–23.
16. Sadler TW. Embryology of neural tube development. Am J Med Genet C Semin Med Genet 2005;135C:2–8.
17. Padmanabhan R. Etiology, pathogenesis and prevention of neural tube defects. Congenit Anom 2006;26:55–67.
18. Song RB, Glass EN, Kent M, et al. Surgical correction of a sacral meningomyelocele in a dog. J Am Anim Hosp Assoc 2014;50:436–43.
19. Huisinga M, Reinacher M, Nagel S, et al. Anencephaly in a German shepherd dog. Vet Pathol 2010;47:948–51.
20. Copp AJ, Brook FA. Does lumbosacral spina bifida arise by failure of neural folding or by defective canalisation? J Med Genet 1989;26:160–6.
21. Fingeroth JM, Johnson GC, Burt JK, et al. Neuroradiographic diagnosis and surgical repair of tethered cord syndrome in an English Bulldog with spina bifida and myeloschisis. J Am Vet Med Assoc 1989;194:1300–2.
22. Arias MVB, Marcasso RA, Margalho FN, et al. Spina bifida in three dogs. Braz J Vet Pathol 2008;1:64–9.
23. Parker AJ, Park RD, Byerly CS, et al. Spina bifida with protrusion of spinal cord tissue in a dog. J Am Vet Med Assoc 1973;163:158–60.
24. Parker AJ, Byerly CS. Meningomyelocele in a dog. Vet Pathol 1973;10:266–73.
25. Clayton HM, Boyd JS. Spina bifida in a German shepherd puppy. Vet Rec 1983; 112:13–5.
26. Lei Y, Zhu H, Yang W, et al. Identification of novel CELSR1 mutations in spina bifida. PLoS One 2014;9:e92207.
27. Bayri Y, Soylemez B, Seker A, et al. Neural tube defect family with recessive trait linked to chromosome 9q21.12-21.31. Childs Nerv Syst 2015;31:1367–70.
28. Berry RJ, Li Z, Erickson JD, et al. Prevention of neural-tube defects with folic acid in China. China-US collaborative project for neural tube defect prevention. N Engl J Med 1999;341:1485–90.
29. Osterhues A, Ali NS, Michels KB. The role of folic acid fortification in neural tube defects: a review. Crit Rev Food Sci Nutr 2013;53:1180–90.
30. Scott FW, de Lahunta A, Schultz RD, et al. Teratogenesis in cats associated with griseofulvin therapy. Teratology 1975;11:79–86.
31. Khera KS, Roberts G, Trivett G, et al. A teratogenicity study on hydroxyurea and diphenylhydantoin in cats. Teratology 1979;20:447–52.
32. Khera KS. Teratogenic effects of methylmercury in the cat: note on the use of this species as a model for teratogenicity studies. Teratology 1973;8: 293–304.

33. Shamir M, Rochkind S, Johnston D. Surgical treatment of tethered cord syndrome in a dog with myelomeningocele. Vet Rec 2001;148:755–6.
34. Clark L, Carlisle CH. Spina bifida with syringomyelia and meningocele in a short-tailed cat. Aust Vet J 1975;51:392–4.
35. Hall JA, Fettman MJ, Ingram JT. Sodium chloride depletion in a cat with fistulated meningomyelocele. J Am Vet Med Assoc 1988;192:1445–8.
36. Plummer S, Bunch SE, Khoo SH, et al. Tethered spinal cord and an intradural lipoma associated with a meningocele in a Manx-type cat. J Am Vet Med Assoc 1993;203:1159–61.
37. James CC, Lassman LP, Tomlinson BE. Congenital anomalies of the lower spine and spinal cord in Manx cats. J Pathol 1969;97:269–76.
38. Platt S, Olby N. BSAVA manual of canine and feline neurology. 4th edition. New York: John Wiley and Sons; 2013.
39. The Cat Fanciers' Association, Inc. Manx show standard. Available at: www.cfa.org/Portals/0/documents/breeds/standards/manx.pdf. Accessed August 11, 2015.
40. De Decker S, Gregori T, Kenny PJ, et al. Tethered cord syndrome associated with a thickened filum terminale in a dog. J Vet Intern Med 2015;29:405–9.
41. Furneaux RW, Doige CE, Kaye MM. Syringomyelia and spina bifida occulta in a Samoyed dog. Can Vet J 1973;14:317–21.
42. Samuelson ML, Dennis SM. Cleft palate associated with meningocele in a pup. Vet Rec 1979;104:436.
43. Ricci E, Bherubini GB, Jakovljevic S, et al. MRI findings, surgical treatment and follow-up of a myelomeningocele with tethered spinal cord syndrome in a cat. J Feline Med Surg 2011;13:467–72.
44. Godzik J, Ravindra VM, Ray WZ, et al. Primary repair of open neural tube defect in adulthood: case example and review of management strategies. Spine J 2015. http://dx.doi.org/10.1016/j.spinee.2015.07.463.
45. Rintoul NE, Sutton LN, Hubbard AM, et al. A new look at myelomeningoceles: functional level, vertebral level, shunting, and the implications for fetal intervention. Pediatrics 2002;109:409–13.
46. Worley G, Schuster JM, Oakes WJ. Survival at 5 years of a cohort of newborn infants with myelomeningocele. Dev Med Child Neurol 1996;38:816–22.
47. Martínez-Lage JF, Ñiguez BF, Almagro MJ, et al. Foreign body reactions causing spinal cord tethering: a case-based update. Childs Nerv Syst 2010;26:601–6.
48. Adzick NS. Fetal surgery for spina bifida: past present, future. Semin Pediatr Surg 2013;22:10–7.
49. Adzick NS, Thom EA, Spong CY, et al. A randomized trial of prenatal versus postnatal repair of myelomeningocele. N Engl J Med 2011;364:993–1004.

Index

Note: Page numbers of article titles are in **boldface** type.

Vet Clin Small Anim 46 (2016) 347–353
http://dx.doi.org/10.1016/S0195-5616(15)00196-5
0195-5616/16/$ – see front matter © 2016 Elsevier Inc. All rights reserved.

vetsmall.theclinics.com

Moving?

Make sure your subscription moves with you!

To notify us of your new address, find your **Clinics Account Number** (located on your mailing label above your name), and contact customer service at:

Email: journalscustomerservice-usa@elsevier.com

800-654-2452 (subscribers in the U.S. & Canada)
314-447-8871 (subscribers outside of the U.S. & Canada)

Fax number: 314-447-8029

Elsevier Health Sciences Division
Subscription Customer Service
3251 Riverport Lane
Maryland Heights, MO 63043

*To ensure uninterrupted delivery of your subscription, please notify us at least 4 weeks in advance of move.

CPI Antony Rowe
Chippenham, UK
2017-01-20 17:56